Practical Epidemiology

Practical Epidemiology

Using Epidemiology to Support Primary Health Care

J PATRICK VAUGHAN

Professor Emeritus in Epidemiology and Public Health, London School of Hygiene and Tropical Medicine, London, United Kingdom

CESAR VICTORA

Emeritus Professor of Epidemiology, Federal University of Pelotas, Brazil

A MUSHTAQUE R CHOWDHURY

Clinical Professor of Population and Family Health, Columbia University, New York

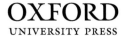

OXFORD
UNIVERSITY PRESS

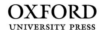

OXFORD
UNIVERSITY PRESS

Great Clarendon Street, Oxford, OX2 6DP,
United Kingdom

Oxford University Press is a department of the University of Oxford.
It furthers the University's objective of excellence in research, scholarship,
and education by publishing worldwide. Oxford is a registered trade mark of
Oxford University Press in the UK and in certain other countries

Published in the United States of America by Oxford University Press
198 Madison Avenue, New York, NY 10016, United States of America

British Library Cataloguing in Publication Data
Data available

Library of Congress Control Number: 2021944884

ISBN 978–0–19–284874–1

DOI: 10.1093/med/9780192848741.001.0001

Printed and bound by
CPI Group (UK) Ltd, Croydon, CR0 4YY

Oxford University Press makes no representation, express or implied, that the
drug dosages in this book are correct. Readers must therefore always check
the product information and clinical procedures with the most up-to-date
published product information and data sheets provided by the manufacturers
and the most recent codes of conduct and safety regulations. The authors and
the publishers do not accept responsibility or legal liability for any errors in the
text or for the misuse or misapplication of material in this work. Except where
otherwise stated, drug dosages and recommendations are for the non-pregnant
adult who is not breast-feeding

Links to third party websites are provided by Oxford in good faith and
for information only. Oxford disclaims any responsibility for the materials
contained in any third party website referenced in this work.

Preface

This book was written during 2020 and 2021 as the Covid-19 epidemic spread around the world and became a global pandemic. The authors experienced several periods of lockdown in their own countries and this cartoon captures many of our experiences as we wrote and edited this book.

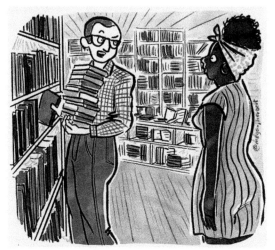

*'We moved a few things around. Travel books are
in the Fantasy section, Politics is in Sci-Fi, and
Epidemiology is in Self-Help. Good luck.'*

With permission of Megan J Herbert (@meganjherbert)

Acknowledgements

In 1989 the World Health Organization (WHO), Geneva, published the *Manual of Epidemiology for District Health Management*, edited by Professor J Patrick Vaughan (London School of Hygiene and Tropical Medicine, UK) and Professor Richard H Morrow (UNDP/World Bank/WHO Special Programme for Research and Training in Tropical Diseases, World Health Organization, Geneva).

The *Manual* focused on the use of epidemiology by health workers in low- and middle-income countries (LMIC). It proved to be very successful and was widely distributed through WHO Geneva and its regional and country offices. The *Manual* was subsequently also translated into several languages, including French, Indonesian, Japanese, Portuguese, Spanish, and Turkish.

In 2002 the two authors, J Patrick Vaughan and Richard Morrow, started to revise and enlarge the scope of the *Manual* and we were joined by George Pariyo of WHO Geneva when we met at the Rockefeller Centre in Bellagio, Italy, as we started planning the revisions. We made excellent progress when in 2005 Richard Morrow returned to the Johns Hopkins School of Public Health, Baltimore when soon afterwards he very sadly suddenly became unwell and died unexpectedly. The revisions were put aside and unfortunately the partially revised manual was never completed nor published. We wish to acknowledge in full all the hard work and writing that all three authors achieved at this time to revise and update the original text.

Starting in late 2019 as the Covid-19 global epidemic started to spread around the world, we decided to revise, update, and rewrite the complete original text and to focus this book on the practical uses of epidemiology to support primary health care in LMICs. In particular, we wanted to focus on the needs of health workers in local and district health systems since they have a crucial role in supporting primary health care and national health developments.

We wish to acknowledge with many thanks the World Health Organization's permission to reproduce many of the original figures and diagrams used in the *Manual of Epidemiology for District Health Management*, published by the World Health Organization in 1989.

Contents

List of Illustrations

Figures

Tables

Boxes

List of Abbreviations

AIDs	acquired immunodeficiency syndrome
BMI	Body Mass Index
CBR	crude birth rate
CDR	crude death rate
CHWs	Community Health Workers
CIOMS	Council for International Organizations of Medical Sciences
COXPH	Cox Proportional Hazards survival analysis
DALYs	Disability-Adjusted Life Years
DHS	demographic and health surveys
DMA	day moving average
DOTS	directly observed treatment short course
DPT	diphtheria–pertussis–tetanus
DSMB	Data Safety and Monitoring Board
EPI	Expanded Programme on Immunization
FGD	focus group discussions
FR	fertility rate
GDP	gross domestic product
GPS	geographical positioning systems
HeaLYs	Healthy Life Years
HIV	human immunodeficiency virus
HPD	hand-held portable device
ICD	International Classification of Diseases
IMCI	Integrated Management of Childhood Illnesses
IMR	infant mortality rate
KM	Kaplan–Meier
LBW	low birth weight
LHMT	local health management team
LMICs	low- and middle-income countries
MDGs	Millennium Development Goals
MICs	multiple indicator cluster surveys
MMR	maternal mortality rate
MOH	Ministry of Health
PCR	polymerase chain reaction
PHC	primary health care
PPE	personal protective equipment
REC	Research Ethics Committee
SARS	severe acute respiratory syndrome

SARSCoV	SARS coronavirus
SD	standard deviation
SDGs	Sustainable Development Goals
STIs	sexually transmitted infections
TB	tuberculosis
TBAs	traditional birth attendants
TFR	total fertility rate
U5M	under-five years mortality
UHC	Universal Health Coverage
UN	United Nations
UNESCO	United Nations Educational, Scientific and Cultural Organization
USD	US dollars
WHO	World Health Organization

About the Authors

J Patrick Vaughan, CBE, MD, FRCP Edinburgh
Professor Emeritus in Epidemiology and Public Health at the London School of Hygiene and Tropical Medicine, United Kingdom.

He has had an extensive career in international health and in health systems planning, evaluation, and research, mainly in low- and middle-income countries. He has worked with the World Health Organization in Geneva, the World Bank in Washington, DC, and as consultant in public health to the UK National Health Service (NHS) in London. He has lived in Papua New Guinea where he worked in government health services, in Tanzania where he helped start the new medical school in Dar es Salaam, and in Bangladesh as research director in public health at the ICDDRB (International Centre for Diarrhoeal Disease Research), Dhaka. He has published many scientific papers and ten books. He graduated in medicine from Guy's Hospital Medical School, London.

Cesar Victora, MD, PhD
Cesar Victora is Emeritus Professor of Epidemiology at the Federal University of Pelotas in Brazil.

He leads the International Center for Equity in Health. Since obtaining his PhD at the University of London in 1983 he has conducted research in maternal and child health and nutrition, birth cohort studies, inequalities in health, and on the evaluation of major health programmes in many countries. He was President of the International Epidemiological Association (2011–14) and won the Canada Gairdner Global Health Award in 2017. He is a highly cited researcher according to the Web of Science 2018, 2019, and 2020.

A Mushtaque R Chowdhury, MSc, PhD
Mushtaque Chowdhury is Clinical Professor of Population and Family Health at Columbia University in New York.

He was the founding Dean of the James P Grant BRAC School of Public Health in Dhaka, Bangladesh, and formerly Executive Director and Vice Chair of BRAC, the world's largest NGO. He was a MacArthur Fellow at Harvard University and spent four years as Senior Adviser to the Rockefeller Foundation, based out of Bangkok, Thailand. He has published nearly 200 articles in national and international peer reviewed journals, including a recent article in the *Oxford Research Encyclopedia*. In 2017 he received the Medical Excellence Award from the Ronald McDonald House Charities of the United States. He is the immediate past President of the Asia-Pacific Action Alliance on Human Resources for Health (AAAH).

Introduction

We focus on the importance of using epidemiological concepts and skills needed to investigate, plan, and deliver primary health care services and to strengthen district level public health programmes. We illustrate these with examples from Low- and Middle-Income Countries (LMICs) and for a hypothetical district population of 200,000 people.

Chapter 1 Epidemiology and Primary Health Care. This outlines the importance of the UN's Sustainable Development Goals (SDGs) and the World Health Organization's principles for Universal Health Coverage (UHC) and the role of district health systems in supporting primary health care.

Chapters 2 and 3 Epidemiological Principles and Population Demography. These explain the use of basic epidemiological and demographic concepts and methods to measure health status and in creating the health information used in planning district services and public health programmes.

Chapters 4 and 5 on Health Information, Reporting, and Surveillance. These describe sources and types of health information and the local reporting and surveillance systems involved.

Chapter 6 on Outbreaks and Epidemics. This explains the dynamics and transmission of communicable diseases and the different kinds of outbreaks and epidemics. The investigation and control of local outbreaks and larger epidemics is briefly explained, including for the Covid-19 global pandemic.

Chapters 7, 8, and 9 on Using Qualitative Methods, Health Surveys, and Quantitative Studies. These present methods for obtaining health data and information, and the advantages and disadvantages of qualitative investigations, health surveys, and quantitative research studies.

Chapter 10 on Organizing Investigations and Surveys. This outlines the importance of obtaining good-quality data through well-organized pilot studies, investigations, and surveys, and the need for specialist expertise.

Chapter 11 on Data Processing and Computing. This explains the steps involved in processing quantitative data obtained from surveys and studies, and the statistical methods used to present the summarized information.

Chapters 12 and 13 on Presenting and Communicating Health Information. These show ways these can be performed and the use of figures, tables, and charts to show visual information.

Chapters 14 and 15 on Epidemiology for Health Planning, Monitoring, and Evaluation. These show how epidemiological methods can be used to strengthen district health planning in support of primary health care and to monitor and evaluate progress towards improving access to health services and public health programmes, as well as their quality and population coverage.

Chapter 16 on Using Ethical Principles. This considers the ethical principles required for the safety and autonomy of individuals and the many ethical issues when planning to tackle health inequalities in district populations.

Chapter 17 on the ABC of Definitions and Terms. These are valid for this publication but different definitions may be used in other contexts. The definitions and terms presented here are based mainly on *A Dictionary of Epidemiology*, 6th edition, edited for the International Epidemiological Association by Miquel Porta and published by Oxford University Press in 2014.

1

Epidemiology and Primary Health Care

1.1 Sustainable Development Goals (SDGs)

The 2030 Agenda for Sustainable Development was adopted by all United Nations (UN) Member States in 2015. There are 17 Sustainable Development Goals (SDGs) that were agreed by all high-, middle-, and low-income countries (previously referred to as developed and developing countries) that aim to end poverty by adopting strategies to improve health and education, reduce inequality, and spur on economic growth while at the same time also tackling climate and environmental changes. The SDGs build on the earlier eight global Millennium Development Goals (MDGs) that aimed to reduce extreme poverty by 2015.

The SDGs address the global challenges of poverty, inequality, climate change, environmental degradation, peace, and justice. All UN Member States have also agreed to try to achieve Universal Health Coverage (UHC) by 2030, as part of the SDGs. The UN Forum on Sustainable Development follows up and reviews progress of the SDGs each year.

SDG 3 is the Health Goal—'Good Health and Well-being: Ensure healthy lives and promote well-being for all at all ages'. This goal puts UHC and access to quality health care at the centre of SDG 3 as a significant contributor to and a beneficiary of sustainable development (Figure 1.1).

Achieving SDG 3 also depends on progress with other health-related SDGs, including those for poverty reduction, education, nutrition, gender equality, sustainable energy, and safer cities. SDG 3 is also related to all other 16 goals, particularly those aimed at ending poverty, achieving zero hunger, ensuring healthy lives, high-quality education, gender equality, and access to clean water and sanitation.

In support of the SDGs the UN quoted the following global health-related information. At least half of the world's population do not have full coverage of essential health services; about 100 million people live in extreme poverty (defined as living on 1.90 USD or less a day) because they also have to pay for

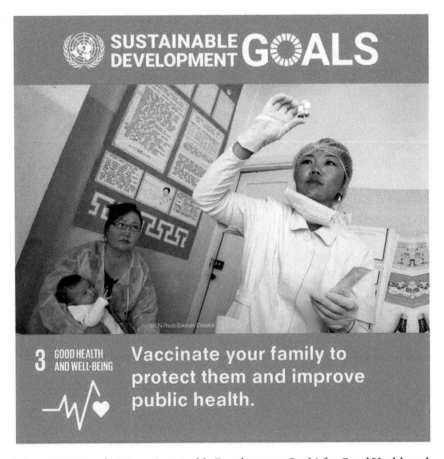

Figure 1.1 United Nations Sustainable Development Goal 3 for Good Health and Well-Being

health care; and about 12% (about 930 million people) of the global population spend at least 10% of their household budgets paying for health care. These 2015 statistics have certainly become even more challenging in face of the global economic effects of the Covid-19 pandemic.

For more details on the SDGs related to health see: www.un.org/sustainabledevelopment

1.2 Universal Health Coverage (UHC)

UHC means that all individuals and communities should receive the health services they need without suffering financial hardship. This includes the full range of high-quality interventions for health promotion, disease prevention, clinical care, rehabilitation, and palliative care. Achieving UHC is one of the targets the UN agreed when adopting the SDGs in 2015.

UHC should enable everyone to access services that address the most significant causes of disease and death and ensure that the quality of those services improves people's health. Good health helps people escape from poverty and provides a basis for long-term economic development.

UHC recognizes and includes:

- All components of the health system: health service delivery systems, health workforce, health facilities, communications networks, health technologies, information systems, quality assurance mechanisms, and governance and legislation
- Individual treatment services and population-based public health programmes
- A minimum package of health services and programmes
- A progressive expansion over time in the coverage of health services and programmes
- Greater financial protection for people as more resources become available

Epidemiological concepts and skills are critical if countries are to make progress towards UHC by strengthening their health systems and improving the coverage of their health services and programmes. This mainly depends on primary health care workers delivering high-quality services and public health programmes, better use of quality management, and good health information systems. All these are essential.

1.3 Health equity and inequalities

Equity in health—health equity—aims to ensure that access to health services and public health programmes is fair and impartial for all people nationally as well as for all people living in districts. It is important, therefore, to analyse health information for any **inequalities**. Achieving greater health equity is a most important ethical priority for district health services and programmes which should be available and accessible to all people living in the district. In addition, equity and fairness are important and health staff should not discriminate against any one on the basis of their age, gender, sexual orientation, ethnicity, religion, disability, socio-economic status, or geographical location.

Promoting greater health equity is difficult and requires that good-quality local health information is available to show the existing inequalities and whether disadvantaged people have full or only partial access to services and programmes. It is important to ask who is included and who is being excluded?

Achieving greater equity involves providing:

- High-quality clinical services and public health programmes that are available to everyone
- Delivery of both clinical and public health programmes to all local communities in the district
- Access to all services for everyone within a reasonable distance and at an affordable cost
- High coverage levels are achieved for priority interventions for all people who need them

Fair health financing also includes the goal that resources and facilities are fairly distributed between:

- curative and preventive services
- urban, peri-urban, and more remote areas
- supporting services and the costs of administration and management

It is very important that any service fees and costs should be locally and socially appropriate and affordable by all individuals. Wasteful health care expenditure should be avoided!

1.4 What is primary health care?

Primary health care is an approach to health and well-being centred on the needs and circumstances of individuals, families, and communities by focusing on their physical, mental, and social health. Primary health care ensures that people receive comprehensive health care as close as possible to where they live. Primary health care is the most efficient and cost-effective way to achieve UHC. Primary health care includes:

- Empowering individuals, families, and communities to advocate and support health policies that protect people's well-being through comprehensive health services and public health programmes
- Ensuring that health problems are addressed through comprehensive promotive, preventive, curative, rehabilitative, and palliative care throughout people's life course
- Placing individuals, families, and the population at the centre of integrated services that use evidence-based public health interventions
- Addressing the broader social, economic, and environmental determinants of people's health

The SDGs and UHC are national-level priorities and they form a framework for regional, district, and local health planning. District health systems have responsibility, therefore, to support SDG 3 by delivering high-quality and accessible local health services and public health programmes. District health teams need to improve everyone's health actively. This will require many more health workers by 2030, particularly in the low- and middle-income countries (LMICs), as well as long-term investments in their education and training.

1.5 Decentralization and local health services

As a part of strengthening the health sector many countries have expanded primary health care services to underserved urban and rural communities. Some countries have reduced or abolished public subsidies and have also reduced or abolished user fees. Another trend has been to decentralize decision-making for local planning and resource allocation to districts, including some being given powers to raise local revenues. Reforms may also include plans for better cooperation between government, non-government, and private health care providers. Some reforms have involved extending private insurance and strengthening community financing schemes.

Central government usually retains control over national matters, such as national health policies, strategic planning, service guidelines, and producing national health information. Ministries of Health usually also retain overall responsibility for national public health programmes such as for tuberculosis, HIV/AIDS (human immunodeficiency virus/ acquired immunodeficiency syndrome), and maternal and child health.

Decentralization can provide a framework for health sector reforms, depending on the powers and authority given to districts by central governments. However, while decentralization has advantages it can also lead to increased inequalities between districts due to inadequate systems for allocating funds fairly between different districts together with a lack of skilled managerial staff in poorer districts.

Decentralization within a Ministry of Health structure, called *deconcentration*, can include more responsibilities for districts in local management, while decentralization by *delegation* happens when other agencies, such as non-governmental organizations (NGOs), are contracted and funded to deliver some essential services on behalf of the Ministry. *Devolution* occurs when full responsibility for planning, resource allocation, and implementation of services is actively transferred to districts themselves. This may involve central government making lump sum allocations to districts so they can determine their own budgetary allocations to different sectors. In other cases, decentralization can involve outright *privatization* where responsibilities are directly contracted out to private not-for-profit and for-profit groups, such as NGOs and private practitioners, clinics, and hospitals.

Districts are an important level for local government planning, with authority often entrusted to a local administration or council of elected or appointed community leaders. Local communities can also be involved in decision-making with representation through local councils, and on governing boards of hospitals and other health care facilities.

1.6 Districts and local health services

Most countries have a local unit of government, often called a district, that has comprehensive powers and local responsibility for implementing national health policies, services, and programmes. Districts provide for the convergence and meeting of local 'bottom-up' community-based planning and services and the 'top-down' development policies of the central government. Districts are the natural level where national policies, strategies, and priorities can be harmonized and integrated to serve the needs of the local community.

Districts often have a population of between 100,000 and 500,000 people and may vary in size from 5,000 to about 50,000 square kilometres. These units are called by various names, such as *upazila* in Bangladesh, *município* in Brazil, county in China, block in India, and district in Kenya. The administrative health headquarters is usually in the main district town where other government offices are also located, such as those for home affairs, agriculture, education, and social welfare.

Districts are usually closely involved in the implementation of local primary health care services and disease-control programmes. They are the key level for planning, managing, and evaluating local health plans, services, and programmes which are usually directed and coordinated by a local health management team (LHMT). How districts are organized varies from country to country and even from district to district. In some countries governments also rely on the services of NGOs and private medical practitioners, clinics, and hospitals. These may or may not be closely linked with government health services. In some countries these are self-contained and operate separately, according to their own priorities. The proportion of health services delivered by the public and private providers varies markedly from country to country. Local health teams play an important role in facilitating their coordination towards improvements in district health services and programmes.

1.7 District health management teams

The local health office is at the centre of a network of health-related activities and facilities that extend from village level to the main district town. These are known as 'bottom-up' or grassroots health activities. All health team members need skills in epidemiology and public health. Teams often consist of the director of district health services and other senior health staff such as doctors, nurses, hospital superintendent, nutritionists, and those in charge of health information, family planning, health education, and environmental services. Some teams also include community representatives. Epidemiology helps to do this and Figure 1.2 summarizes the district situation in many countries.

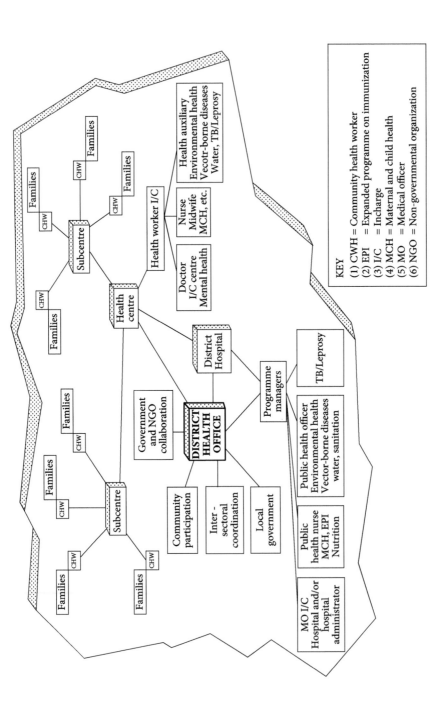

Figure 1.2 Central role of the district health office in a local health system

Reproduced with permission from Vaughan, J Patrick, Morrow, Richard H, and World Health Organization, Manual of epidemiology for district health management, World Health Organization; Geneva, Switzerland, Copyright © 1989

'Top-down' government planning includes national development policies, strategies and health plans, standards, and guidelines. These guide districts in their efforts to plan and implement high-quality management of local health care services and public health programmes. District teams are responsible for planning and managing all their day-to-day health-related activities. It is essential that the team is concerned with the health of all people living in the district and not just those who attend the services.

Local health teams must first ensure that health services and programmes are **delivered** to everyone in the district so that they all people have **access** to comprehensive health care performed to nationally accepted standards of care, whether the services are provided by government, NGOs, or the private sector. Finally, the services and programmes also need to provide **high-quality** services and that health programmes achieve high **coverage** for the prioritized national interventions that people need.

In determining which health interventions have high priority, the notion of 'value for money' is useful—the amount of healthy life gained by each intervention provided per currency unit expended, together with how equitably the gains will be distributed among the population. The chapters entitled Epidemiological Principles (Chapter 2), Population Demography (Chapter 3), Planning and Management (Chapter 14), and Monitoring and Evaluation (Chapter 15) provide further details.

1.8 Epidemiology and district planning

Epidemiology is concerned with whole populations and is an essential discipline as countries adopt health policies and strategies based on agreed and effective interventions to improve health outcomes. Its concepts and methods are central to health planning and management for assessing the effectiveness of health interventions, for analysing their equitable and fair distribution, and for forecasting future health needs.

Epidemiology is also critical for improving the planning of district health services that need to focus on the needs of all patients, families, and communities. Local health services and programmes rely on using evidence-based interventions to do the 'right thing in the right way at the right time'. This means using evidence-based interventions and guidelines for health promotion, prevention of health risks, clinical care, disease control, rehabilitation, and palliative care.

Epidemiology also aims to promote greater **equity**, reduce **inequalities**, and enable the fair allocation and distribution of scarce health resources based on all people's health needs. Epidemiology is crucial for planning and implementing local primary health care and public health programmes, including for any marginalized and vulnerable people.

Everyone in the district population should benefit from the health interventions and services. Priority needs to be given first to achieving the fair **delivery** and distribution of health facilities and staff, as well as achieve high levels of population **access** to good services. These must also be of high **quality**. Delivery, access, and high-quality interventions are all needed if high population **coverage** is to be achieved for all the most important health interventions. These four concepts are essential if primary health care is to be successfully implemented by local health planning and management teams.

Epidemiology also promotes greater **equity** and the fair allocation and distribution of scarce health resources based on all people's health needs, including for well-planned local primary health care and public health programmes for marginal and vulnerable people.

The local health team headquarters and district hospital are usually a major centre for all health-related activities. High-priority health services commonly include those for chronic and lifestyle-related diseases, such as cardiovascular diseases and diabetes, preventive health programmes such as immunization and family planning, and environmental provision of safe water, housing, and waste disposal. Other health priorities are programmes for women and children, control of communicable diseases, and health promotion for better lifestyles and reducing behavioural risks by improving nutrition, encouraging physical fitness, and providing services for mental health.

> **What are the main responsibilities of local health management teams**

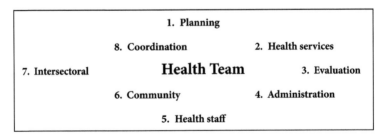

Figure 1.3 Essential responsibilities of the local health management team

The district health team's essential planning and management responsibilities include:

1. Monitoring compliance with national interventions, programmes, guidelines, and standards
2. Provision of public health services, including health education, supervision of health care services
3. Evaluation and monitoring of all health interventions for delivery, access, quality, and coverage
4. Collecting and analysing health information for local services and programmes
5. Health administration of budgets and finances, drugs and vaccines, transport, equipment and supplies, and medical wastage
6. Workforce planning, in-service training, supervision of health staff and community-based workers
7. Community involvement, including with local government and non-government agencies
8. Coordination between all government and non-government health service providers in the district
9. Intersectoral collaboration, including with agriculture, education, water, and environment
10. Local governance for public transparency and financial accountability

These responsibilities involve the following main activities:

- Annual district health planning in keeping with national policies and plans
- Implementing the local plan for priority programmes and coordinating with all district providers
- Organizing services, including hospitals, health centres, and community health workers
- Budgeting for the plan, with records and financial controls for disbursement of funds
- Management support for transport, supplies, staff training, supervision, and information systems
- Collecting and evaluating health information to measure progress towards plan objectives

1.9 Making a public health diagnosis

Figure 1.4 and Table 1.1 summarize the similarity in approach between clinical care and public health. The clinician examines individual patients and assesses the pathological significance of clinical symptoms and signs in order to make a differential diagnosis. After taking the patient's history and performing a physical examination, laboratory and special tests can be ordered to confirm the specific diagnosis, which is followed by prescribing the appropriate treatments and advice.

In public health, epidemiological skills are essential for collecting and examining health information about the whole population and selecting suitable indicators that describe and explain the health problems in the district. Next it is necessary to make a public health diagnosis and to decide which of the national programmes would be most effective in improving the health status of the whole population and any particular at-risk sub-groups. If the data from the routine health information system are not sufficient, the health team may need to investigate by using qualitative assessments or conduct health surveys or even special quantitative studies.

However, there is a fundamental and very important difference between the two approaches. Clinicians see patients after the onset of a health problem or disease, and treatment does little to reduce the number of new cases of the

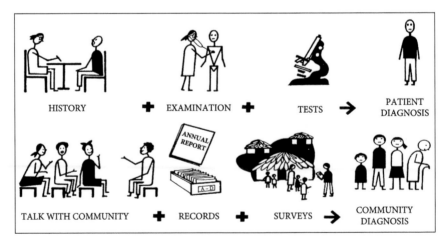

Figure 1.4 Comparing clinical medicine and public health

Reproduced with permission from Vaughan, J Patrick, Morrow, Richard H, and World Health Organization, Manual of epidemiology for district health management, World Health Organization; Geneva, Switzerland, Copyright © 1989

Table 1.1 Comparing clinical medicine and public health approaches

	Clinical medicine	Public health
1. Objective	Caring for patients with diseases	Improve health status of the whole population
2. Information needs	Clinical history, physical examination, laboratory investigations	Population data, analysis of disease patterns, special studies, and health surveys
3. Diagnosis	Case history, differential diagnosis, and probable diagnosis	Population diagnosis and public health priorities for action
4. Action plan	Patient investigations, treatment, follow-up, and rehabilitation	Priority health interventions, services, and programmes delivered and accessed
5. Evaluation	Patient follow-up and assessment of cure	Improvements in equity, delivery, access, quality, and coverage to improve health status for all

disease in the wider population. Clinical services do not remove the underlying causes of such health problems in the population.

Epidemiology and public health attempt to understand why new cases of the health risk or disease keep occurring and how control programmes can reduce the incidence of new cases. Although epidemiology is a fundamental skill for all health personnel, it is particularly directed at the prevention and control of diseases where evidence-based health interventions can achieve improvements in the population's health status.

1.10 Health information needs

Local health teams have responsibility for organizing both curative care services and the public health programmes (see Figure 1.5).

The 'iceberg' phenomenon shows that most people attend the curative health services because they are ill, while for the intervention programmes people need to be persuaded to attend for their own future benefit. Health data from these two different services can be linked together and are complementary.

How health information is collected varies from country to country. Some countries publish information for individual districts while in others the information exists but is scattered among various different ministries, agencies, or NGOs. Most countries have routine information systems to collect data

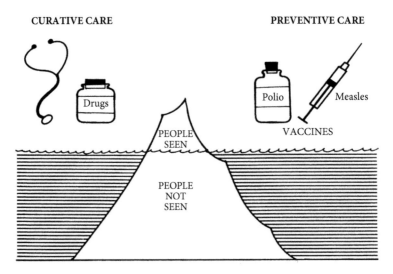

Figure 1.5 Health teams are responsible for both clinical and public health services

Reproduced with permission from Vaughan, J Patrick, Morrow, Richard H, and World Health Organization, Manual of epidemiology for district health management, World Health Organization; Geneva, Switzerland, Copyright © 1989

from health facilities that are collated at district level and then forwarded to the Ministry of Health or a national statistical agency.

Using health information requires a good knowledge of the local district population and the total number of people who need both health services and programmes. For instance, how many pregnancies occur each year in the district and who delivers the babies? What proportion of deliveries are supervised by a trained health worker? How many young children suffer acute illnesses and what proportion are fully vaccinated? What percentage of households have access to a safe water source or a latrine?

The health information listed in Box 1.1 helps to provide answers to these questions.

Additional data may also be collected through surveillance systems and surveys for specific health problems and epidemic diseases. Qualitative assessments and special investigations can be used to understand people's concerns about their own health problems and their perceptions on the quality of local health services. Other information sources include statistical agencies that conduct census, demographic, and other health surveys. Other sectors, such as agriculture and education, non-governmental organizations, and community and religious groups may also collect useful health data.

Box 1.1 Summary of district health information required for local health planning

General information
- History, physical, and climatic characteristics, community organization, economic developments, occupations, organization of local government
- Geographical distribution of villages and towns, major roads, and important features such as rivers, lakes, and mountains
- Relevant cultural practices and health beliefs, social organization of villages and households, main forms of seasonal economic activity and employment
- Literacy, food security, and poverty status of the population

Population
- Size, age/sex structure, geographical distribution, migration patterns, growth rate
- Access to health facilities by distance and travel time

Health status, morbidity, and mortality patterns
- Birth and fertility rates
- Maternal, foetal, infant, child rates, and morbidity and mortality rates
- Common causes of morbidity, mortality, and epidemics
- Main underlying health problems such as food availability, hygiene, housing, water supply, excreta disposal

Health services
- Number and distribution of government, NGO, and private health facilities, personnel, and programmes
- Adequacy of local management support, logistics, and supplies
- Number, distribution and type of health workers and their supervision
- Financial allocations and budgets, recurrent and capital

Health programmes
- Family planning, pregnancy, delivery, newborn and postnatal care
- Infant and child health: growth and nutrition, management of childhood illnesses

- Adolescent health
- Immunization
- Environmental health: water supplies, excreta disposal, and hygiene
- Communicable disease control: respiratory, diarrhoea, HIV/AIDS, malaria, Covid-19
- Non-communicable: heart disease, diabetes, hypertension, accidents/injuries
- Control of infectious diseases, local outbreaks, epidemics, emergencies
- Domestic violence, mental health, accidents, and injuries

Many countries have carried out large-scale **demographic and health surveys** (DHS) and **multiple indicator cluster surveys** (MICS) which have collected important data for planning. However, these are often limited by the small average sample number of sub-national areas that are surveyed in DHS and MICS. On average, nine areas per country are sampled and these are usually large states or provinces and not districts, due to sample size limitations. Thus few national surveys are representative at district level. Some specific programmes, such as immunizations and nutrition, may carry out sample surveys for knowledge, practice, and coverage to provide detailed information on the health of infants, children, and mothers. Some of these use survey methods such as the so-called 30-Cluster surveys. In addition, most countries conduct a **census** every ten years that provide specific data and indicators on the entire national population, and some may also provide this information for individual districts.

These various sources of information can be invaluable for district data and even sub-district information but health teams may then have to collect their own information. However, in some countries health information, particularly maps, census data, demographic and vital statistics are not collected routinely nor are readily available in a form that is useful at the local level.

1.11 Systems approach to health planning

Local planning starts by using national policies and guidelines to organize the district's priority services and public health programmes which will be supported by centrally allocated staff, finances, and other resources.

Local planning can be summarized as a series of steps starting from the national planning level towards achieving local impact, as follows:

- **Policies and strategies** formulated for national planning
- **Deliver** local interventions as clinical services and public health programmes
- **Access** to facilities improved by the locally delivered services and programmes
- **Quality** of delivered services improved
- **Coverage** improved for population based programmes
- **Impact** achieved for disease reduction and improved health status

Epidemiology is essential for implementing this systems approach and for the necessary local management and planning. Epidemiology is also essential for measuring changes in health status and for evaluating progress.

The systems approach divides the local planning process into five main stages as shown in the box below. This starts with **inputs** from the national plans that provide a framework for the local level planning **processes** that are organized to **deliver** the necessary district interventions. When these are successful they **achieve** positive health **outcomes** and finally **impact** on the local population's health status.

INPUTS	PROCESSES	OUTPUTS	OUTCOMES	IMPACTS
Plan	Organize	Deliver	Achieve	Evaluate
National health policies and plans	Allocate staff finances and resources	Implement plans for services and programmes	Interventions delivered for access, quality, and coverage	Achievements for impact on health status and diseases

1.12 Epidemiology and the health planning cycle

This cycle starts with a detailed knowledge of the local district population and the available health resources with the aim of organizing health care services and public health programmes that lead to improvements in health status for everyone in the local population (see Figure 1.6). High priority has to be given to improving the **delivery, access, quality**, and **coverage** of both health services

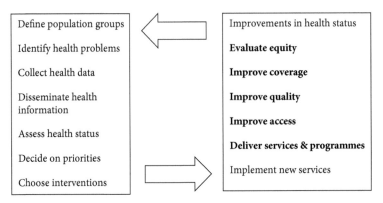

Figure 1.6 Epidemiological skills are required in the circular planning cycle

and public health programmes. Epidemiology is a vital skill for measuring these indicators.

Delivery of services and programmes is the first step in making sure that all priority health interventions are being planned and organized for the benefit of the whole of the local population.

Access measures the proportion of the district's population that has a particular health facility within reasonable reach, which is commonly measured by distance (5 km or 10 km) and/or time (1–2 hours walking). For access it may also be important to examine costs, social factors, and cultural beliefs.

Quality measures how well the health services and programmes are organized and using nationally accepted and evidence-based international standards and guidelines for health interventions.

Coverage measures the proportion of people or households in the whole district population who are in need of a health intervention or service who have actually received it, such as the percentage of households with a safe water supply or of pregnant women who attend for antenatal care.

Equity helps ensure that access to health services and public health programmes is both fair and impartial for everyone. To achieve better health equity, district health teams must analyse local health information for any inequalities. Achieving greater equity is a most important ethical priority. District health services and programmes should be available and accessible to all people.

Coverage for the whole population will only be high if first the delivery of interventions is well organized and then if access and quality interventions are in place. For example, immunization coverage can remain low if these interventions are not delivered to all children who should have good access to immunizations at health centres, sub-centres, or mobile clinics. If health facilities and staff are not offering good-quality services then high immunization coverage will also not be achieved. For example, coverage might be measured by the percentage of young children who have been immunized with three doses of DPT (diphtheria–pertussis–tetanus) vaccine. If coverage is too low the local health team may then have to rely on introducing new services, such as more mobile clinics and expanding the use of mass vaccination campaigns.

1.13 Ethical principles for primary health care

In planning for primary health care there are four main **ethical principles** that are recognized internationally and which apply in both public and private clinical care services and which are also widely applied in public health programmes. The following ethical principles are covered and explained in more detail in Chapter 16.

Autonomy: It is the right of individuals to be in charge of decisions regarding their own health. This gives priority to informed consent, privacy, confidentiality, and the right of people to access their own health information.

Justice: Aims for a fair and equitable distribution of benefits and risks in the population, including that all people are given equal access to treatment facilities and public health programmes. This also includes fair financing between clinical and public health interventions and between investing in people in different urban and rural geographical locations.

Beneficence: Produce benefits that far outweigh risks in all curative services and public health programmes.

Non-maleficence: Avoid any unnecessary harm to individuals or communities by both personal services and public health programmes.

> ETHICS HELPS PLANNING MAKE FAIRER CHOICES

2

Epidemiological Principles

2.1 Definition and approach

Epidemiology is essential for describing patterns of health and disease in whole populations and detecting any changes that occur over time. It enables the frequency and duration of health risks and diseases to be defined, classified, and counted, together with their consequences for morbidity, mortality, disability, and the burden of disease. The natural history of health status and diseases may change over time and these changes need to be monitored and explained.

Epidemiology helps to understand inequalities and to explain causes, risk factors, and contributing or predisposing conditions that influence equity through the frequency of health problems and diseases. It provides the basis for **interventions** that promote health, prevent disease, cure illness, and rehabilitate patients. It also provides health workers with practical and relevant skills for health planning, management, and evaluation of local health services and programmes.

Definition: Epidemiology is the study of the distribution, frequency, and determinants of health-related problems and diseases in specific human populations. The purpose of epidemiology is to obtain, interpret, and use health information to promote health, prevent disease, and cure and rehabilitate patients.

Epidemiology helps to describe health issues and disease problems or events by answering the following questions:

Who or which people are involved?
When or at what time?
Where or in which place?
What is the 'burden of disease'?
What is the natural history of health risks and diseases?

Epidemiological is useful in four different ways. First is **descriptive epidemiology** which in the above definition is the part concerned with disease distribution and frequency by asking: what is the problem or disease or event and its frequency, who is involved, where, and when?

The second use is called **analytical epidemiology** because it attempts to analyse the causes and determinants of health problems or diseases or events by testing hypotheses to answer such questions as: how is the problem or disease caused, and why is it continuing? This approach looks for statistical associations between possible **exposures** and subsequent health **outcomes.**

The third use is **experimental epidemiology** to test **interventions** in which clinical and population-based controlled trials are used to answer such questions as: what is the efficacy of clinical treatments in curing people? How well do interventions protect people? Do they reduce the incidence of new cases and control diseases?

The fourth use may be called **evaluation epidemiology** because it can be used to measure the effectiveness of different interventions used in health services and programmes, such as health messages for immunizations and how well they are implemented locally and nationally. It also asks:

So what? How effective are the intervention programmes? Have there been any subsequent improvements in health status?

Descriptive and evaluation epidemiology are particularly useful for the planning and analysis of local health services and programmes. Analytical and experimental epidemiology rely on important concepts and methods that usually require specialist expertise to be used successfully. They are mainly used for health and research studies, such as case-control (retrospective) studies, cohort (longitudinal) studies, and controlled trials. These require specialized epidemiological and statistical methods that are suitable for large-scale investigations and research studies.

2.2 Epidemiological information

Classical epidemiology searches for patterns by examining for characteristics of **persons (who), place (where),** and **time (when).** Epidemiology bases all its findings and uses on well-defined populations or groups of people. It also provides important information for planning, managing, and evaluating all local health activities based on particular local populations. Epidemiology also helps to plan both clinical services and public health programmes that promote health and prevent, cure, and control diseases. The key descriptive data necessary for this information can be approached through a series of questions:

What is the health problem, disease, condition, or event and what is its frequency, manifestations, and characteristics?

Who is affected, with reference to such variables as age, sex, socio-economic status, ethnic group, occupation, heredity, risk factors, and health behaviours?

Where does the problem or condition occur, such as at home or near place of residence or work, its geographical distribution, and place of exposure?

When does it happen, in terms of time, such as which days, months, seasons, and years? Is it increasing or decreasing over time?

Why does the health problem, disease, condition, or event occur and what is its association with different exposures, such as to risk behaviours, sources of infection, or environmental factors?

What are the interventions and programmes that could make a difference when implemented?

It is important that health workers base their work on the needs of the **total population** as well as on any specific high-risk sub-groups, such as mothers, children, and the elderly. This requires demographic and health data on the total population as well as information on sub-groups, such as people who attend the health services and programmes. Non-attenders are important because they are often different from the people who do attend.

A most important epidemiological concept is the total population at risk, called the **denominator population,** for a health problem or service or health intervention. This information is needed for health planning, management, and evaluation of services and programmes. It is also required to estimate indicators of delivery, access, quality, and coverage when evaluating all health intervention programmes.

Delivery of services and programmes is the first step in making sure that all priority health interventions are being planned and organized for the whole of the local population.

Access measures the proportion of the district's population that has a particular health facility or clinic or intervention within reasonable reach.

Quality measures how well health services and programmes are being implemented using the recommended standards and guidelines.

Coverage measures the proportion of people or households in need of a health service or facility who have actually received it.

Achieving high values for these four indicators is the single most important task for local health teams. Assessing delivery, access, quality, and coverage are essential starting points for making improvements in local health programmes.

For example, to know the coverage of immunization—an intervention—it is important to know the total number of children who actually received their immunisations compared to the total number of children needing immunization in the population. What proportion actually received their immunizations? Similarly what proportion of all known cancer or tuberculosis patients are actually attending for treatment, or what proportion of all houses in need of insecticide spraying have actually been sprayed?

WHAT POPULATION COVERAGE IS BEING ACHIEVED?

2.3 Descriptive epidemiology

Classical epidemiology searches for patterns by examining characteristics of **persons or who, place or where,** and **time or when.** The first stage in understanding a health or disease problem or event is to look for patterns by describing it with the epidemiology characteristics or variables of Who? Where? and When? (see Figure 2.1). With all the information assembled, the next stage is to explain all the known facts. How can the frequency—**incidence or prevalence**—and **distribution** of new cases be explained?

Who or People? Some important variables are age, sex, education, occupation, income, health behaviours, cultural and religious group, family size, nutritional state, and immune status. Other characteristics might be clinic attenders and non-attenders, households with and without latrines, and normal and low birth-weight infants. Any relevant variable can be used provided that the subjects can be clearly placed in one category or another.

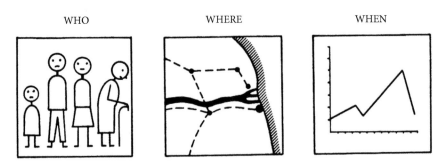

Figure 2.1 Descriptive epidemiology—Who? Where? When?

Reproduced with permission from Vaughan, J Patrick, Morrow, Richard H, and World Health Organization, Manual of epidemiology for district health management, World Health Organization; Geneva, Switzerland, Copyright © 1989

Where or Place? Where people live or work may partly determine which health or disease problems they suffer from and what use they make of the available health services. For example, variables might be:

- Town, village, or isolated dwelling
- High or low altitude
- Proximity to rivers, forests, animals, factories, or use of toxic substances
- Distance from the local clinic, health centre, or local hospital

When or Time? It is important to know when health problems are most common and when is the greatest incidence of new cases. New cases, episodes, or events may be analysed by hour, day, week, month, year, or decade. The time period depends on what is being analysed, for instance:

- New cases of cholera diagnosed per day
- New cases of measles per week
- New pregnant mothers registered per month
- New cases of cancer diagnosed in one year
- New cases of rare diseases diagnosed in a decade

2.4 Measuring frequency

Incidence and **prevalence** are the two main measures of frequency for health problems, diseases, and intervention events, including for the measurement of the use of health services and programmes. However, it is very important to be clear on their differences and on which measure is being used.

Incidence measures the number of **new** cases, episodes, or events occurring in a defined population over a defined **period of time**, such a week, month, or year. Incidence is the most basic measure of frequency and is the indicator that shows whether a condition is increasing, decreasing, or remaining the same within the population. It is the best measure to use in research studies of health interventions, in the management of services, and in surveillance systems to evaluate disease control programmes.

Incidence is the best measure for short duration diseases such as measles, diarrhoea, pneumonia, or accidents. Other incidence examples include deaths occurring in a district in one year, new cases of HIV/AIDS diagnosed per year, number of new women attending for antenatal services for the first time per year, and the number of new patients diagnosed with a cancer or stroke in one year.

The term 'incidence' is often used in its broad sense but incidence in populations can be either a rate (incidence density) or a risk measure (cumulative incidence). Advanced epidemiology uses the term 'rate' to express the incidence of disease or episodes, for example in 100 or 1,000 persons, and expresses their full-time risk as being over months, years, or even over a lifetime. The term 'rate' expresses incidence of disease for say 1,000 persons-years at risk and it expresses a proportion in which the numerator is part of the denominator.

Person-time incidence rate measures incidence in a population at risk over longer time periods and is divided by the number of person-time units, such as years observed for the period, to give the incidence rate. This measure is often used in cancer studies, such as for new cases of carcinoma of the uterus and cervix, or for the duration of life following treatment. The cumulative (lifetime) incidence at the individual level is also a risk measure, rather than a rate, such as the lifetime risk of developing breast cancer or coronary heart attacks.

INCIDENCE MEASURES ALL NEW CASES DURING A DEFINED TIME PERIOD

Prevalence measures the total number of **existing** cases, episodes, or events occurring at **one point in time**, commonly on a particular day. Prevalence is often used for chronic conditions like physical disabilities and mental health. Prevalence is more complicated to interpret than incidence because it depends upon the number of people who have developed their illness in the past and who continue to be ill at the point in time. It is a combination of the previous incidence of a condition and its average duration for how long it lasts.

The term 'prevalence rate' is often used, although strictly speaking prevalence measures are proportions rather than rates in their strict sense (as defined earlier under incidence rates).

Examples of using prevalence include the number of tuberculosis patients on a register at the beginning of each month divided by the total population, or the proportion of all hospital beds occupied per day.

Surveillance systems that report new cases rely on measuring incidence, such as for new cases of yellow fever and for maternal deaths. Cross-sectional surveys generally provide prevalence data.

> **PREVALENCE MEASURES ALL CASES AT ONE POINT IN TIME**

Under stable conditions, incidence and prevalence are related by the following formula:

$$\text{Prevalence} = \text{incidence} \times \text{average duration of the condition}$$

For conditions with a long average duration, such as most cancers or tuberculosis, incidence is lower than the prevalence. For example, the prevalence of pulmonary tuberculosis in countries with weak control programmes is commonly between 0.5% and 1.0% or 5–10 patients per 1,000 population per year and the average duration for untreated illness may be about 4–5 years. This means that incidence is about a quarter of prevalence or 0.1–0.2% or 1–2 new cases per 1,000 people per year.

In countries with effective tuberculosis control programmes, good diagnostic services, and reporting systems the incidence of new cases of tuberculosis may be closer to prevalence because the average duration of the disease is shorter due to cases receiving effective treatment. Countries that do not have such good information systems commonly rely on reporting prevalence data.

2.5 Using numbers and rates

Incidence and prevalence data are used in reporting health information and may be given as whole numbers or presented as rates.

The most readily available data will often be **absolute numbers**. For instance, these are used in monitoring important infectious disease outbreaks, such as cholera and Ebola, when the populations are still stable and restricted in locality and time. Reports on the delivery of health services often also use whole numbers as these indicate the service load, for example the number of patients seen in antenatal clinics and for road traffic accidents seen by accident and emergency services. Both incidence and prevalence numbers are used in reporting health information but they can also be given as calculated rates rather than whole numbers.

Using whole numbers can lead to false conclusions when examining for **trends over time** or when comparing the frequency of diseases in different **populations** or communities. For trends and comparisons it is best to use incidence and prevalence rates. If the population size and age-sex structure differ or has changed over time it is best to use **age-sex specific rates or standardization** before these groups are compared (see Annex One).

It is also important to be clear whether the rates are being calculated for cases, episodes, or events. Rates depend on using the **population at risk,** the group of people in which these cases, episodes, or events may arise. This population is also the target population that might benefit from a programme of interventions, such as all children in the district for child health services and all women aged 45+ years for screening of breast cancer.

The total number of cases, counted as people, episodes, or attendances, is called the **numerator** and the total target population at risk is the **denominator.** All people in the denominator must be, by definition, be at risk of becoming a part of the numerator population. Each rate must have the time period or date attached to it. The term rate is often used to express a proportion in which the numerator is part of the denominator.

Numerator = number of people, episodes, or events
Denominator = total population at risk
All rates should state the time and the factor

Incidence rate—This is the fundamental measure of frequency in epidemiology and is a direct measure of risk for new events in a population. In a dynamic population the denominator can also be the estimated population at the mid-period of a year. For everyone in the denominator it must be possible for them to become part of the numerator. For example, for prostate cancer the denominator at-risk population includes only men and new cases in one year period gives the annual incidence rate. For some common diseases, such as diarrhoea that may occur more than once in the same person, the incidence rate can be expressed as episodes per child per year which may be equal to 2.5 or 3.0 episodes per child per year.

Epidemiology also discriminates between two types of incidence measures. The first uses incidence rate as the number of new cases divided by person-time at risk, with the estimated mid-year population being a good estimate of the number of persons at risk during that year. The second measure is cumulative incidence (or incidence risk), which is the number of people who developed the condition during the year divided by the at-risk population at the beginning of the same year. However, except for a few common diseases, the rate and risk are very similar.

Prevalence rate (proportion)—This is the ratio of the total number of cases or individuals who have a risk or disease or who are experiencing an event at a particular point of time, compared to the total population at risk of having that event at this point in time. It is a measure of current status. For many chronic diseases prevalence rates are often more available than incidence rates.
Incidence and prevalence rates are defined as follows:

$$\text{Incidence} = \frac{\text{New cases in specified period of time}}{\text{Total population at risk}} \times \text{factor}$$

$$\text{Prevalence} = \frac{\text{Existing cases at specified point in time}}{\text{Total population at risk}} \times \text{factor}$$

All rates are multiplied by a factor chosen to present the rate as a whole number. Common factors are 100, 1,000, and 10,000.

Example 1: In a district with a mid-year population of 200,000, there are 40 new cases of hypertension reported in one year:

$$\text{Incidence of hypertension} = \frac{40}{200,00} \times 1,000 = 0.2 \, \text{cases}/1,000 \, \text{Population}$$

This rate is the same as 0.02 cases/100 people or 2.0 cases/10,000 people

Example 2: In a district with a mid-year population of 200,000, there are 150 tuberculosis cases on the local disease register on 1 January.

$$\text{Prevalence of tuberculosis} = \frac{150}{200,00} \times 1,000 = 0.75 \, \text{cases}/1,000 \, \text{Population}$$

This rate is the same as 0.075 cases/100 people or 7.5 cases/10,000 people on 1 January.

Age- and sex-specific rates for incidence and prevalence are used to present findings separately by age groups and for men and women. These rates can also be used to compare events in different populations. For age- and sex-specific rates the denominator includes only those people in the particular age/sex groups. For example, for the age-specific fertility rate for women aged 20–24 years the denominator is all females in the population in the age group 20–24 years. It is important to use the appropriate denominator in all calculations.

In estimating prevalence of a communicable disease the denominator used should be the total number of individuals at risk of contracting or diagnosed with the disease. In a sample survey this would be all the individuals in the specific age-sex grouping. For instance, in estimating the malaria prevalence of *Plasmodium falciparum* in blood slides, the denominator should be the total number of people from whom slides were taken and then read.

2.6 People, episodes, or attendances?

It is extremely important to be clear about what is being counted. For instance, are the **cases** made up by counting people or episodes or attendances? For shorter duration illnesses such as common cold and diarrhoea a person may have more than one attack in one year and may attend a clinic more than once. For longer duration illnesses like cancer or tuberculosis, patients may be counted as one episode but have attended clinics every month and 12 times over the past year.

To estimate the proportion of the population sick at any one point in time and suffering a longer duration chronic illness—its prevalence—it is the total number of sick people.

To evaluate the effectiveness of a malaria control programme, data is needed on the number of new cases—incidence—detected commonly in one month or in one year.

To study the use of health services it is preferable to have separate data for both new attenders and separately for their repeat attendances. It is best if clinical record data show new consultations separately from repeat consultations.

WHAT IS BEING COUNTED? PEOPLE, EPISODES, OR ATTENDANCES?

2.7 Case definitions

Good case definitions are essential in assessing the outcomes of intervention programmes and for deciding whether or not the number of cases is changing, increasing, or decreasing, such as for health risk behaviours or diseases. Clear diagnostic criteria are needed to distinguish all cases from non-cases. Case definitions are very important when using both incidence and prevalence measures.

Sometimes the case definition requires a spectrum, such as **non-cases and possible, probable, and definite cases** with laboratory confirmation (see Figure 2.2). For example, people living in a malaria-endemic area with fever, headache, and body aches may be diagnosed with malaria and treated.

The Ministry of Health, however, might only count those cases confirmed by a positive blood slide. During the 2020 Covid-19 pandemic the use of different diagnostic criteria in different countries has made international comparisons of incidence and death rates very complex and potentially misleading.

2.8 Making use of rates

There are two main reasons for using rates rather than whole numbers. First rates are necessary when making comparisons, for example when comparing the local population today with that ten years ago or between two different populations at the same time. Both situations may have different numbers of people at risk and different population age-sex structures. This requires

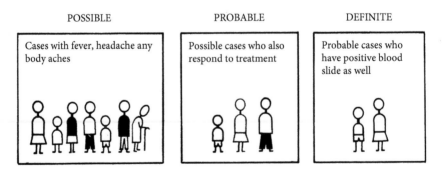

Figure 2.2 Diagnostic criteria for possible, probable, and definite cases of malaria

Reproduced with permission from Vaughan, J Patrick, Morrow, Richard H, and World Health Organization, Manual of epidemiology for district health management, World Health Organization; Geneva, Switzerland, Copyright © 1989

standardising for the populations. This can be achieved by using **age-sex-specific rates** or **population standardization** (see Annex One). These two methods can be used to make valid comparisons over time or between several different districts at the same point in time.

Secondly, rates are also useful for calculating the number of **expected cases or events**. This is often best done using known rates published by a national statistical bureau. However, due to the wide variations between different districts it may be best to use data from another local source of reliable rates, such as another similar district. Local data may be incomplete or even outdated but national level rates are an average that can hide considerable geographic and socio-economic inequalities within a country and between districts. Wide variations can even exist between what appears to be similar areas.

It is often best, therefore, to use reliable incidence and prevalence rates from another similar local setting. It is most important that local health teams use the best of the known rates to calculate expected cases and these will usually be more accurate than those calculated from the district's own local data. For instance, if the national prevalence for leprosy is 1 per 100 people or the infant mortality rate is 80 per 1,000 infants per year, the approximate number of expected cases occurring in one year can be calculated.

To understand the importance of **disease severity** it is necessary to assess its frequency as well as it being a cause of disability and death. Mortality is a major indicator of a population's health status and can be used to understand and measure the burden of disease. For instance, stillbirth and perinatal mortality rates are useful indicators for the quality of obstetric care services and neonatal and infant mortality rates are often used as proxy indicators of child health and overall development in low- and middle-income countries (LMICs).

Mortality rates are a form of incidence and expressed as the number of deaths in a defined population during a defined time period usually one year. The rate can be calculated for total deaths, for age- and/or sex-specific deaths, for all cause-specific deaths, and for disease-specific morbidity and mortality.

Another indicator of severity is case fatality which is the number of deaths divided by the number of people who have suffered from the disease. For example, case fatality for Covid-19 has been estimated to be less than 1.0% to over 3.0%, depending on the setting. The difference between mortality and case fatality rates is in the denominators: the total population is for mortality and reported cases for case fatality. Case fatality rates are always higher than mortality rates. However, when testing for a disease that is widespread, more cases will often be reported which can show up as a case fatality compared to situations in which fewer individuals are tested and diagnosed. It is incorrect to report case-fatality rates as being mortality rates.

Composite measures such as Healthy Life Years (HeaLYs) and Disability-Adjusted Life Years (DALYs) combine frequency, morbidity, disability, and mortality into one measure. However, they are not suitable for small geographical areas like districts because of the numerous assumptions behind these metrics that make them unreliable in small area populations. These metrics are useful for individual countries with large populations and for making global estimates.

These composite measures can be used to prioritize national health services, allocate scarce health resources, examine equity of health status, and evaluate health interventions and programmes. The amount of HeaLYs gained from health-related interventions can be compared with the costs of implementing them to give estimates of **cost-effectiveness**. Resources can then be allocated to interventions that will produce the largest gain in healthy life per unit of expenditure, but it is important to consider the distribution of any gains and whether they are both equitable and fair.

2.9 Health status indicators

Useful basic indicators of health status can be grouped in to four main categories:

- Risk factors
- Nutrition
- Morbidity
- Mortality

Risk factors are mainly identified as threats to health and some are antecedent causes for possible later morbidity and mortality. For example, they may be lifestyle behaviours such as for smoking, alcohol intake, lack of exercise, obesity, unprotected sex, and mental depression. Environment risk factors for poor health include low income, unemployment, substandard housing, contaminated water supplies, and lack of latrines. Some so-called **risk markers** are associated with health outcomes but are not themselves causal factors for subsequent ill health.

Nutritional status is a risk factor and an underlying causal condition for ill health in both under-nutrition and over-nutrition. For instance, low birth weight (LBW)—less than 2500 grams—as a percentage of all newborn babies and anthropometric measurements are commonly used for assessing the nutrition status of infants and young children, including weight-for-age, height-for-age, and mid-upper-arm circumference. Health status is indicated by the percent of children classified as having mild, moderate, and severe malnutrition according to Z-scores.

Malnutrition includes both under- and over-weight and obesity. These are measured by the Body Mass Index (BMI), defined as the person's weight in kilograms divided by their height squared in metres. Overweight is defined as a BMI of 25–29.9 and for obesity it is over 30.

Morbidity indicators are usually based on disease-specific incidence and prevalence rates for common and/or severe diseases, such as the common cold, strokes, and cancers. Another way to assess morbidity is to list the overall top ten most common causes of ill health or for more severe illness the top ten diagnoses for hospital admissions. A more accurate way is to analyse the individual disease rates for each major age/sex group separately.

Mortality indicators are mainly the crude mortality for all ages and case fatality rates for specific disease episodes. A more accurate method is to calculate rates for age-sex specific groups, stillbirths, neonatal, infant and child mortality, maternal mortality, expectation of life at birth, and disease-specific age/sex mortality rates.

For many LMICs, a short list of local basic health status indicators might include:

- Behavioural and socio-economic risk factors
- Fertility
- Life expectancy at birth
- Neonatal and infant mortality
- Child mortality in the 1–4 age group
- Maternal mortality
- Nutritional status
- Main causes of morbidity
- Main causes of mortality

More details on these health status indicators are given in Chapter 3 on demography and in Chapter 4 on epidemiological health information.

WHICH POPULATION GROUPS ARE AT HIGHER RISK?

3

Population Demography

3.1 Demographic and epidemiological transitions

A thorough understanding of the demography of populations is essential when using epidemiology. As countries undergo economic and social development, they can experience sharp declines in mortality followed much later by a reduction in fertility. **Demographic transition** refers to a population moving from high birth rates balanced by high death rates and little or no population growth to a population with continuing high birth rates but falling mortality levels, especially in the under-five age group. This leads to rapid **population growth**. Demographic transition contributes to an increase in life expectancy and a change in the dependency ratio, with fewer children per household, a higher proportion of the elderly, and an increase in single person households.

Later there is a fall in **fertility** and the lower number of births leads to lower and more stable birth and death rates. Population growth is also lower and there is a gradual increase in the proportion of elderly people. The **population pyramid** moves from a wide base reflecting the large proportion of children to a narrower base and with nearly equal percentages in all age groups (see Figure 3.1). The proportion of people in the elderly age groups will gradually expand over decades compared to younger age groups.

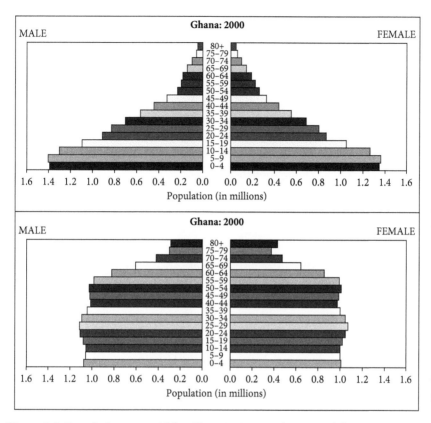

Figure 3.1 Population pyramid for Ghana in 2000 and projected for 2050
Source data from US Census Bureau, International Database

Countries that have undergone economic development usually experience a fall in under-fives mortality, mainly due to reductions in malnutrition and communicable diseases. Lower fertility eventually occurs and this leads to reductions in mortality. Some countries may then experience negative growth which can then lead to them promoting pro-natalist policies. For instance, Sweden's population has gradually been falling and China has abandoned its one child policy.

Reductions in **maternal mortality** usually occur more slowly and mainly when economic and social development, communications, and health services become more advanced.

Epidemiological transition is associated with the demographic transition and causes a changing pattern of diseases, from earlier high levels of infectious diseases and high levels of childhood mortality to an increasingly elderly population who live longer and suffer more from chronic non-communicable diseases such as diabetes, raised blood pressure, strokes, and cancers.

3.2 District population

Although the demographic and epidemiological transitions happen slowly it is important that local health teams have recent and reliable data on the district population and its health problems.

Many countries perform a national **population census** every ten years, based on information collected by enumerators who visit every household in small enumeration areas. They collect information on all people living in a household on a particular day and the figures are combined to give the total population data for the whole district. These are further aggregated to provide national figures which are published as census reports which are usually available at local and national government offices.

Table 3.1 shows a typical population by age groups for a low- to middle-income country (LMIC). Many countries publish this information. Infants (< 1 year) commonly make up about 2–4% of the total population, children 0–4 years about 15–20% and those 0–14 years about 40–44%. Women in the reproductive age range (15–44 years) are often about 20% or one-fifth of the local population.

It is important to know the percentage of the population in each of the district's different age groups. If local figures are not available, census reports will usually show the percentage figures. These can be used to determine the approximate number of at-risk people in the main age groups in local districts (see Table 3.1).

Table 3.1 Approximate population by age groups for a typical district in a low-income country

Age group (years) male and female	Percentage	Approximate district population
< 1 year	4%	8,000
1–4	14%	28,000
5–14	26%	52,000
15–44	43%	86,000
45–64	10%	20,000
65 +	3%	6,000
All ages	100%	200,000

Table 3.2 Approximate ratio of people in selected age and sex groups in a LMIC population

Infants	0–11 months	1 in 25 people
Young children	0–4 years	1 in 5 people
All children	0–14 years	2 in 5 people
Women of child bearing age	5–44 years	1 in 5 people
Women 15–44 years + children	0–4 years	2 in 5 people

For population-based public health programmes an important group are children under five years old and women in the reproductive age group 15–44 years. Children under five years (about 18%) and women aged 15–44 years (about 20%) make up about 40% or two in five people in the district.

For local health planning and management, the approximate number of people in selected groups, particularly children and women aged 15–44 years, can be seen in Table 3.2.

3.3 Population pyramids

Figure 3.1 presents the population pyramid for Ghana in 2000 and that projected for 2050. Population pyramids also provide useful estimates for denominators (the at-risk population) when calculating certain age- and sex-specific rates.

There may be differences between men and women in the same age group because both women and men may be either under- or even over-counted. For example, men are more likely to migrate from rural to urban areas and to work in towns, near factories, mines, and on plantations, which can result in an apparent higher proportion of children, women, and the elderly. Conversely, women in rural areas may be reluctant to be counted or be absent and away attending to farm crops and livestock when the count is undertaken.

As the demographic transition continues to occur the pyramid becomes broader in the older age groups. This change is largely determined by changes in the population's fertility levels and less by changes in the levels of mortality. It has been predicted that as population fertility continues to decline, pyramids will eventually over many decades reverse and become broader in the older age groups and narrower in the younger age groups.

The age-sex structure for the total population can be presented by a **population pyramid**, using the percentage of males and females in each five-year age group.

3.4 Population density

The average number of people per square kilometre (km^2) is a measure of **population density**. This varies within districts and is usually higher near large towns, areas with fertile land, and close to roads and rivers. If the local population rapidly increases or decreases, recent migration is the most likely explanation. Some districts have over 1,000 people per km^2, particularly in Asia, while some areas in Latin America and Africa often have fewer than 50 people per km^2 (180 people per square mile).

Knowledge of population density and distribution is important when planning district health services, particularly when planning to improve the delivery of services and planning for better access to community health workers and clinics, health sub-centres, and health centres. Distance affects people's access to local facilities and higher distances can lead to lower population coverage by health programmes.

3.5 Demographic rates

Rates are important indicators of preventable deaths, for example from malnutrition and infectious diseases which are common in the one to four years age group. Because local health information systems are usually inadequate for accurate calculations, many rates are calculated from censuses and special surveys. Table 3.3 below summarizes some important numbers and rates.

Table 3.3 Number of births and deaths in an LMIC district population of 200,000 people

Rate	Rate / 1,000	Events per year	Events per week
CBR	20–40 / 1,000	Live births 4,000–8,000	Live 80–155
CDR	10–20 / 1,000	Deaths 2000 –4,000	Child deaths 40–80
IMR	40–150 / 1,000	Infant deaths 240–1250	Infant deaths 5–25
MMR	1–5 / 1,000	Maternal deaths 4–45	Maternal deaths < 1 / week

Crude birth rate (CBR)

This is usually estimated from the census or special demographic surveys and is given by this formula:

$$\text{CBR} = \frac{\text{total births in one year}}{\text{total mid-year population }\left(\text{all ages, same year}\right)} \times 1000$$

In high-fertility countries, the CBR may be around 40–45 births per 1,000 people per year, and in lower fertility populations it may be lower at about 15–20 births per 1,000 people per year. Official census figures are often available for individual districts and by applying them to its population it is possible to estimate the total number of births expected each year. For example, in a district of 200,000 people with a CBR of 40 births per 1,000 the expected births are 8,000 per year, or an average of about 150 per week. It is important, however, to note that the number of births can vary in different seasons and some months may have a larger number of births than the average. This is important when making plans for local services.

$$\text{Total births} = \frac{\text{CBR}}{1,000} \times \text{population} \quad 40 \times \frac{200,000}{1,000} = 8,000 \text{ births per year}$$

If the district health information system reports that trained health workers attended an average of about 100 births each week, obstetrical coverage can be estimated to be 52 × 100 ÷ 8,000 = 65% of all births. This suggests that obstetrical coverage is too low and needs more attention.

Fertility rate (FR)

This age-sex specific rate—usually derived from the census or special demographic surveys—measures how frequently women in the reproductive age range (15–44 years) are having babies. This rate is calculated by dividing the number of births in a year by the mid-year total number of women in the appropriate age group. If the CBR is high the fertility rate will also be high. In LMICs the average annual fertility rate may be about 100–150 births per 1,000 women aged 15–44 years and around 200 in high-fertility populations and 30–60 in lower fertility populations.

The **total fertility rate** (TFR) is the average total number of children born by all women in the population by the end of their reproductive age of 15–44 years. It is the aggregate of all the age-specific fertility rates. In a stable population with no increase or decrease this rate is often just more that an average of two births per woman. This is the population replacement rate. The TFR is commonly about five in many LMICs while it can be as high as seven to ten in some poorer populations and less than one in some more economically advanced countries.

Crude death rate (CDR)

This rate is not standardized for the population's age-sex structure and is calculated as follows:

$$CDR = \frac{\text{total number of deaths in one year}}{\text{total midyear population }(\text{all ages, same year})} \times 1,000$$

The CDR commonly ranges from around 10 deaths per 1,000 people per year in more highly developed countries to 20 deaths or more per 1,000 per year in many LMICs.

Infant mortality rate (IMR)

The IMR is commonly seen as a good general measure of health status and also of socio-economic development. It is usually calculated from the census or special demographic surveys. Local estimates based on locally reported data are unreliable unless there is a good vital registration system.

The IMR is the proportion of all live born babies who die before their first birthday.

$$IMR = \frac{\text{number of deaths among infants }(\text{aged} < 1 \text{ year})\text{ during one year}}{\text{number of live births during the same year}} \times 1,000$$

In high income countries the IMR is about 10 per 1,000 and in LMIC it can be about 100 or even higher. The IMR is a population average rate which can vary for different seasons and months. The actual rate is often higher in rural areas and for poor and disadvantaged groups and it is usually lower in the wealthier groups and for urban people. The total number of expected infant deaths can be calculated as follows:

$$\text{Expected number of infant deaths} = \frac{\text{IMR}}{1,000} \times \text{no. of births}$$

For example, in a district with a population of 200,000 and 8,000 births per year and an IMR of 100, the estimated number of infant deaths would be:

$$\text{Number of infant deaths} = \frac{100 \times 8,000}{1,000}$$
$$= 800 \text{ per year, or about 15 deaths per week}$$

Perinatal and neonatal mortality rates

The perinatal mortality rate includes both foetal deaths and deaths occurring in the first week of life, expressed as per 1,000 live births. A stillbirth is the death of a foetus weighing 500 g or more, or of 22-weeks gestation or more if its birth weight is not available (ICD 10).

Early neonatal mortality is the death of a live newborn in the first seven days of life and neonatal mortality are deaths occurring during the first month of life. Neonatal mortality is the number of deaths in those babies aged 28 days or less in one year and expressed as neonatal deaths per 1,000 live births during this same period of time.

Child mortality rate (CMR or under-five mortality rate)

This is the annual number of deaths in the 0–4 age group per 1,000 live births, averaged over the previous five years. It is equivalent to all deaths in the 0–4 age group in a year divided by the total population in that age group.

Child death rate

This is based on deaths between 1–4 years old per 1,000 children in this age group. This rate is usually derived from a census or special DHS (demographic and health surveys) as it is more difficult to obtain than that for the CMR.

Maternal mortality ratio (MMR)

This ratio (rate) covers all deaths directly related to and caused by pregnancy and during delivery and in the post-partum period. In many low income countries this rate can be 100–500 or more maternal deaths per 100,000 live-births, compared to about $5-10 \div 100,000$ in many high income countries.

$$MMR = \frac{\text{Pregnancy-related maternal deaths in one year}}{\text{Number of live births in the same year}} \times 100,000$$

In a district with 200,000 people and a CBR of 40 per 1,000, about 8,000 live births might be expected per year. If the district's MMR is 100–500 per 100,000 live births (the same as 1–5 deaths per 1000 live births), there could be 8 to 40 maternal deaths per year or less than 1 per week in the district. Due to the small number of maternal deaths in a district, it is often best to use whole numbers rather than the ratio.

The MMR is a fundamental indicator of health and development and shows the largest differential between low- and high-income countries (LMICs) of any health indicator. The ratio gives a misleading impression of the risk to mothers as it uses births as the denominator rather than the number of women at risk in the child-bearing age group. A MMR of $100 \div 100,000$ in Africa compares to about $5 \div 100,000$ in Europe (20 times greater) but because the average number of births per woman is much higher in Africa their actual lifetime risk of dying may be up to about 80 times greater or even more.

3.6 Life expectancy

Life expectancy at birth, also known as **expectation of life**, is the average number of years a newborn baby can be expected to live if the current mortality trends were to continue unchanged. It is an average that is determined mainly by mortality in the first years of life and it is, therefore, lower in many LMICs due to high levels of infant and child mortality. It is often used as a measure of current health status and mortality conditions as well as an indication of general socio-economic development. In some LMICs, death rates for girls and women may be higher than for boys and men in most age groups.

Demographic **life tables** can be used to calculate the future life expectancy for any age or sex group as the number of years that individuals can expect to live. Expected years of life lost from a harmful exposure or treatment is a measure of the loss of years of life experienced by those exposed to a harmful exposure compared to those not exposed.

3.7 Population growth

This depends on the balance between the annual number of births and migration into the area and the numbers of deaths and migration out of the area (Figure 3.2).

In an urbanized population an increase in growth is usually mainly due to in-migration rather than births substantially outnumbering deaths.

The number of people migrating into or out of a district will probably have to be estimated as accurate figures may only be available from the national census. The average annual increase or decrease in the local population can be estimated when the total population is known at two points in time and by

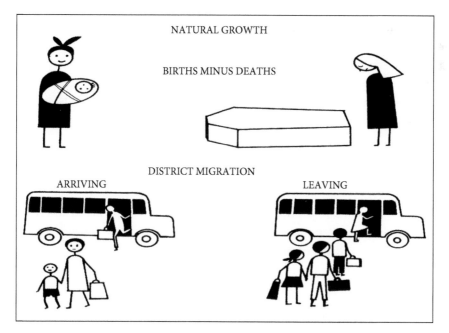

Figure 3.2 Growth in district population due to natural growth and migration
Reproduced with permission from Vaughan, J Patrick, Morrow, Richard H, and World Health Organization, Manual of epidemiology for district health management, World Health Organization; Geneva, Switzerland, Copyright © 1989

dividing the difference by the number of years. Dividing the estimated annual increase (or decrease) by the mid-year population gives the probable population growth rate.

Natural population growth rates exclude migration and they determine how fast the district's population will probably grow as follows: Rate of natural population increase = CBR minus CDR

> **With 1% natural growth the population will double in about 70 years**
> **2% in about 35 years and 3% in about 20–25 years**

3.8 Sources of population information

The number of people in the district and their age, sex, and geographical distribution is necessary for planning, managing, and evaluating the health services, particularly for their delivery and access. This data can be used to provide estimates for the:

- total number of expected live births and deaths per year, and
- number of people at-risk being seen by services and programmes

Data sources include census reports, special studies, Ministry of Health publications, research studies, non-governmental organizations (NGOs), and research units, and, where available, from the vital registration system.

Census Bureau reports

These are the most reliable national figures as they are usually based on a census undertaken every ten years or so. The census publications may include local information for individual districts.

Reports and special studies

Besides health reports, special studies and surveys may also be carried out by other ministries, such as agriculture, education, and rural development. Universities, NGOs, and research units often conduct important socio-economic surveys, and mapping and census data may be collected by national programmes for malaria and other disease control projects, and nutrition and family planning programmes.

Civil registration and vital statistics

Most countries have a system for regularly registering information on births, deaths, marriages, and migration. However, in many LMICs registration data is often incomplete and it is estimated that only about one-third of the world's population is included in any registration system. Some countries have registration based on sampling a small proportion of the country's total population. While vital registration systems can provide good quality information for local planning, it is most important to estimate how incomplete they are.

Other sources

Local authorities for housing, education, law enforcement, and public utilities may have valuable information, and NGOs and faith-based organizations are often well informed and have their own documented data. In addition, national utility and mobile phone companies frequently have large datasets.

Estimating populations

If there are no reliable demographic data on the total population the health team can make a crude estimate by sampling 100 random households and multiplying by the average household size for the district which is often reported by the census. If this is also unknown, an estimate of average household size can be made by visiting every 10th or 20th household in urban settlements or rural villages and asking for details of all residents. Visit 100 households for a crude estimate. The average household size is often about five people in rural areas, although it may be higher or lower in urban areas.

3.9 Accuracy of data

How accurate the data need to be depends on how information will be used in decision-making. Accuracy of population data is often limited by how well it was collected and by the socio-economic, educational, and cultural understanding of the population. To validate household data for child born and their present health status a complete birth or pregnancy history may be required from all woman resident in households starting with the first child born. Long gaps between births can indicate a death as pregnancies often occur about every two years in high fertility populations. Women may be reluctant to speak about a child's death and it may be necessary to ask specific questions discreetly.

Rough estimates will probably be sufficiently adequate for local area planning and resources might be wasted on efforts to obtain more accurate data. The more developed the health services, the greater the need for more detailed and accurate data in management and evaluation.

HOW ACCURATE ARE THE DATA?

Information should be as accurate as reasonably possible, available in good time, and represent good value. It is often neither possible nor necessary to obtain high degrees of accuracy. The aim should be to have data to assist in decision-making.

Age

Age is closely related to local disease patterns and is required for most health reports and studies. People may not know their age in years but may know the year they were born. Where birth records are not available age can be estimated using a calendar of notable events that occurred previously in the community. For example, a person's age might be estimated by asking: 'How many seasons after the last earthquake were you born?'

For young children aged 6–24 months, approximate age can be estimated in months by adding 6+ to the number of erupted teeth, provided the child has not suffered from severe malnutrition.

Many people will give different ages on separate occasions, with older people being more inaccurate. Some say they are about 30 or 40 rather than 32 or 39. Men may wish to seem older and may report their wives as being younger. To reduce such misclassifications 5- and 10-year age intervals can be used, such as 0–4, 5–9, 10–14, 15–24, 25–34, 35–44, 45–54, 55–64, 65+. To reduce this source of error, it is important to document procedures, to use strict criteria when recording age, to specify how age was calculated, and to indicate the sources for the information.

Gender

Survey results may be invalid when there are marked differences between the male/female composition of a population compared to the general population. For example, in some countries it is a common practice for women to stay secluded in their homes and interviews may be very difficult to obtain which can result in women being under-enumerated in censuses. In rural areas in many LMICs, men migrate away for employment. Considerable care is needed to take these differences into account.

Marital status

The precise definition of 'married' or 'separated' varies considerably in LMICs and between different cultures. Local definitions may be required as the concept of marital status and the nuclear family may not reflect local traditions. Understanding the population's customs and lifestyles will help to define this variable.

Ethnicity

Ethnic groups tend to have similar social and cultural practices which can result in either higher or lower disease estimates. It is important to understand socio-cultural patterns as these can provide clues on how diseases may be understood and reduced or controlled.

Occupation

This can be difficult to define when people have multiple daily occupations at the same time or have moved their employment between different occupations. Recording only the present employment can be misleading. It is important, therefore, to record both present and past occupations. For example, a worker may have spent the past 15 years in the mining industry but as a result of pulmonary tuberculosis was unable to continue and then obtained new employment as a night watchman. Rural areas may also have marked seasonal changes in occupation, such as farming during the rains and fishing after the harvest. The possibility of exposure to more than one environmental risk must always be kept in mind.

Other variables

Data on parity, religion, social class, place of residence, and mobility may also be required. Nomads can present issues for censuses and registration systems as their whereabouts may be unknown and data are difficult to record. Data collection methods often need to be adapted to the local context. For example, men may leave their homes early in the morning to work in their fields or to look after cattle, while women may not be permitted to mention their husbands' names or leave their houses if unaccompanied.

3.10 Demographic surveillance

Recording population events is usually done by special demographic and research studies that identify all existing households and map them before a **census enumeration** is undertaken. **Geographical positioning systems** (GPS) can be used to position households and to map physical features such as villages, roads, and rivers. Households can be assigned unique location coordinates. Aerial photography and Google Earth can also be used. Large-scale maps may be necessary for densely populated urban areas and slum settlements.

Surveillance involves collecting detailed household information with an enumeration questionnaire, such as for age, sex, residence, income, and ownership of land and other goods and questions on survivorship, fertility, and mortality. Each individual is usually identified by name and given a unique survey number and geographical location. Mobile phones and hand-held portable devices can be used for collecting data on installed questionnaires and with permission taking photographs of individuals.

For a **census** it is essential to distinguish between residents and visitors and whether the enumeration is using a *de jure* definition of the population, those normally resident in the defined area, or a *de facto* definition for all people in the household on the particular census day.

Census data are based on the date of birth, age, and sex of all individuals, as well as perhaps recording cultural and ethnic group, religion, education, and marital status. Questions may also be asked about survivorship of parents, spouses, and older and younger siblings, and a record of deaths in the household during the previous 12 months for estimates of mortality. Each female aged 15–44 years can be asked questions about the number of live births she has ever had and about whether her most recent live birth is still alive or not. Fertility rates and infant and child mortality rates can be derived from this information. It may also be important to collect information on the use of modern contraception methods.

A similar system can also be used for **epidemiological surveillance** for detecting the incidence of particular diseases and for recording illness episodes within households. Arrangements may be needed to regularly update this information through repeat household visits of not less than once a year and in a demographic and health surveillance (DHS) system they are often carried out once every three to four months.

3.11 Death registration and certification

National censuses usually provide age- and sex-specific mortality rates by regions and districts based on reported causes of death. However, systems for registration of deaths and certification based on the **underlying causes of death** are usually weak in many LMICs and therefore unreliable.

Death registration

This is the official record of a person's death and usually includes name, age, sex, date of death, and address. This may be a legal responsibility of the health system although it is often not well enforced.

Death certification

Death certification records the causes of a person's death as stated by a physician or other responsible health worker. Deaths should be classified by the **underlying cause** although often it is the most direct cause leading to death that is quoted.

Information from death registration and certification can be used to compile mortality statistics and for the surveillance of specific diseases, particularly in countries where registration and certification are reasonably complete. A sudden rise in certified deaths from a particular cause may indicate a serious outbreak and a cause for concern. Well recorded causes of deaths can be used to evaluate the effectiveness of some disease control programmes. Deaths from human immunodeficiency virus/acquired immunodeficiency syndrome (HIV/AIDS) is an example of a disease that is often under-reported.

In some countries sample household surveys are used to provide more reliable mortality estimates when the death registration and certification systems are inadequate. Verbal autopsies can also be used to determine some causes of mortality, particularly when the clinical situation is clear in under-fives for diseases such as neonatal tetanus and severe diarrhoea. Age- and sex-specific mortality profiles provide important information for health planning, management and evaluation.

Certification of the cause-of-death should be based on the **International Classification of Diseases** (ICD) which is widely used for the analysis of hospital in-patient records and which can provide good information on causes of serious morbidity and mortality.

An outline of a typical death certificate is shown in Figure 3.3. Part I of the certificate shows the stated sequence of events beginning with the leading direct cause of death and followed by the underlying cause of death due to disease, injury, or complications. In Part I the death should be recorded by the underlying cause of death, such as (a) coronary heart disease, and with other underlying or antecedent causes given in Part I(b) and (c), such as (b) diabetes and (c) obesity. Separately in Part II, other significant disease conditions are listed, such as chronic obstructive lung disease.

Cause of Death Certificate	Approximate time between onset and death _____
Part I: Disease or condition directly leading to death _____	(a) _____
	due to (or as a consequence of)
Antecedent causes _____	(b) _____
	due to (or as a consequence of)
Morbid conditions, if any, giving rise to the above cause stating the underlying condition last _____	(c) _____
Part II: Other significant conditions contributing to the death, but not related to the disease or condition causing it.	_____

Figure 3.3 Outline of medical certificate of the cause of death

3.12 Population checklist

- On a large-scale district map mark all health facilities, villages, and special features
- Determine the current total population by age and sex and its density in different areas
- Assess in and out migration and note the annual official district growth rate
- Calculate the likely number of people in the 0–11 months and 1–4, 5–14, 15–44, 45–64, and 65+ year age groups and the total number of women aged 15–44 years
- Obtain official figures for the local crude birth rate, crude death rate, perinatal and neonatal rates, infant mortality rate, and maternal mortality ratio
- Calculate the approximate total number of births and deaths expected per week and per year. Do this for all deaths and separately for infant, child, and maternal deaths

4

Epidemiological Health Information

4.1 Important diseases

The most important causes of disability, morbidity, and mortality may be apparent in the data on the health status of the whole population. To plan, manage, and evaluate health services and programmes it is necessary to see which interventions, if well implemented, lead to the greatest health improvement for the available resources.

Locally collected data help to identify priority diseases and **high-risk groups**. Details of national health programmes are included within national policies and plans which guide the planning, management, and evaluation of local health services and programmes.

Four epidemiological factors suggest the importance of a disease:

- **Frequency**—diseases with a high incidence or prevalence
- **Severity**—diseases causing serious disability, are highly infectious, have a high case fatality
- **Interventions**—diseases for which specific and evidence-based interventions are available
- **Epidemic**—diseases that potentially can lead to serious epidemics and a pandemic

Two composite population indicators that combine frequency, disability, morbidity, and mortality in a single measure are **DALYs** (disability adjusted life-years) and **HeaLYs** (healthy life years) (see Section 4.7).

> ### IMPORTANT AND CONTROLABLE DISEASES SHOULD HAVE A HIGH PRIORITY

For example, *Falciparum malaria* can be widespread and have a high **case fatality** in under-five-year-old children, and malnutrition can also have a high prevalence and contribute to high child mortality. Diseases such as cholera, dengue, meningococcal meningitis, severe acute respiratory syndrome (SARS), and Ebola are potentially epidemic and also can have high case-fatality rates.

If effective health intervention programmes are available these should also have a high priority. High-priority interventions are those that are known to be highly effective and that provide the most gain in healthy life for the least expense.

For example, tuberculosis (TB) remains among the top ten leading global causes of death due to infection and, together with HIV (human immunodeficiency virus), cause a high burden of dual infection in many low- and middle-income countries (LIMCs). Globally about a third of the population is infected with *Mycobacterium tuberculosis* although most people are not ill from TB in LIMCs. TB control remains important in the UN Sustainable Development Goals and is a priority for the World Health Organization (WHO).

4.2 Epidemiological information

Local routine **health information systems** usually have information on the frequency and distribution of the locally important and common causes of morbidity and mortality. Mortality data from censuses and special **surveys** are usually more accurate than the data that are routinely reported by the local information system, which may be deficient in both quality and quantity, particularly for illnesses among selected population sub-groups. Several important biases can lead to underestimates, such as low geographical access to health facilities, low use of health care services due to public perceptions about low quality of care, travel costs and fees for clinic attendances and medicines, particularly for poor people. Poor **quality of care** is an important determinant for whether people use services and the public trusts local services and programmes.

Local routine health information systems usually record data on the frequency and distribution of locally important causes of morbidity and mortality but these data are often not presented in a useful way.

While most local health data are based on people attending services, it is very important to also know who and why people are not attending or accessing the services and programmes they need. A helpful analogy is the 'iceberg phenomenon' which illustrates that what is visible is only a fraction of all the people that need the services (see Figure 1.5).

Main sources of morbidity and mortality data

- Censuses
- Out-patient clinic records
- Hospital in-patient records
- Notifications
- Workplace and school records
- Special studies and surveys

Out-patient clinic records

Patients' illnesses are often recorded by symptoms rather than by a diagnosis and clinic attendances are often given as totals rather than separately for new and repeat case totals. Records for attendances at health posts and health centres can provide useful patient data but the information often suffers from selection biases similar to those for hospitals. People most likely to use the services are usually those living near a facility and who can afford the time and pay any fees. Although clinics provide some data on the most frequent symptoms and diseases in the local community, it is less useful for assessing access, quality, or programme coverage.

Hospital in-patient records

Analysis of hospital records can provide some high-quality information on the local causes of serious illnesses, particularly if hospital discharge records use the **International Classification of Disease** (ICD) codes for patient discharges and mortality status (see Box 7.2). However, patient hospital attendances are subject to selection biases similar to those affecting data from primary health care facilities but these biases are usually even more marked for hospitals inpatients.

Disease notifications

Most countries have statutory requirements to report certain diseases that require prompt action by the health authorities, including many infectious diseases. Medical practitioners and other health staff may be legally required to provide such notifications and local environmental health officers are often responsible for this reporting.

School and workplace records

These may provide data based on sickness absences, periodic health examinations, and findings from screening programmes. Data on employed people can be biased due to ill people losing their employment which can lead to a highly selected sample of healthy people. Where school attendance is low the information may be substantially biased towards wealthier children living nearby and against those children who are socially and economically disadvantaged.

Special studies and surveys

Important diseases with a low frequency (incidence or prevalence) can be underestimated when only a few cases show up in poorly functioning health services. Leprosy is a good example. Some illnesses that do not present clear symptoms and signs may also go undetected, such as sub-clinical infections and chronic diseases like diabetes, hypertension, mental ill-health, and eye diseases.

4.3 Morbidity patterns

Infant and childhood morbidities can account for up to a half of all out-patient illness attendances occurring in the younger age groups. Pregnant mothers and children also account for most attendances at preventive programmes held at health centres, health posts, and mobile clinics.

> **ROUTINE INFORMATION SYSTEMS MAINLY REPORT COMMON AND EASILY RECOGNIZED SYMPTOMS AND DISEASES**

For serious morbidities, hospitals and in-patient records provide most of the clinically most reliable data but these must also be interpreted with caution. For instance, in some low-income countries malaria and diarrhoeal diseases alone may account for up to a quarter of all out-patient attendances and a high proportion of in-patient episodes.

The most frequent causes of hospital admissions in a typical LMIC can include:

- One-fifth or 20% of all admissions are for pregnancy, deliveries, and their complications
- One-fifth (20%) of all admissions are for children's illnesses such as malaria, pneumonia, and diarrhoea
- Heart disease, cerebral vascular diseases, strokes, HIV/AIDS, and injuries can utilize a large number of hospital beds due to lengthy individual inpatient stays
- About ten different conditions commonly account for about a half of all hospital admissions

4.4 Mortality patterns

The main causes of mortality differ between countries. Communicable diseases account for nearly half of all deaths in many low income countries but only about 1 in 20 deaths in high-income countries. In LMICs, malnutrition, accidents, and maternal complications are major causes of death, while communicable and non-communicable diseases together account for about two-thirds of all deaths in these countries. In high-income countries, however, non-communicable diseases can account for over 80% of all deaths due, for example, to cancers, cardiovascular disorders, diabetes, and trauma.

The most common causes of death in LMICs, based on crude death rates per 100,000 population, has changed quite significantly over recent decades with a marked increase in the importance of non-communicable diseases. For deaths in LMICs the WHO found in 2016 that the following were the top 10 commonest causes of death, presented here with their approximate crude death rates per 100,000 population in brackets:

- Ischaemic heart disease (125)
- Strokes (60)

- Lower respiratory infections (45)
- Chronic obstructive pulmonary disease (40)
- TB (30)
- Diarrhoeal diseases (30)
- Diabetes mellitus (25)
- Preterm birth complications (25)
- Cirrhosis of the liver (20)
- Road injuries (20)

The WHO estimates that about 10 million people annually become ill with TB and 1.5 million die from TB each year. It is the world's top infectious disease cause of death. About a quarter of the world's population has been infected with TB bacteria but only 5–15% become ill with active TB disease. The rest have TB infection but are not ill. About half of all active TB disease cases are in eight high-burden countries: Bangladesh, China, India, Indonesia, Nigeria, Pakistan, Philippines, and South Africa.

In some low-income countries children may account for up to 40% of all deaths

---

4.5 Expected numbers of cases

It is important for programmes to know what population coverage is being achieved. Coverage is a measure of how many people a programme intervention reaches as a proportion of all those people who actually need it. For instance, high coverage of all pregnant women and newborns needs to be achieved if specific mother and child health promotion and preventive interventions are to be effective. The expected number of people in each category and the actual number seen by the programme should be available to the local health team to calculate programme coverage.

Local health services should estimate the expected number of cases of important diseases or events to assess the extent of coverage with prevention programmes and treatment services. For example, in TB and leprosy control programmes the number of cases expected in a district each year can be estimated through the use of rates derived by national special surveys carried out in sample areas, perhaps every five to ten years.

For instance, if the incidence rate for new cases of pulmonary TB is expected to be 1 per 1,000 people per year, there should be about 200 new cases expected each year in a district population of 200,000. The expected number of newly diagnosed TB cases in one year is:

$$\text{incidence rate} \times 200{,}000 = 0.001 \times 200\ 000$$
$$= 200 \text{ new TB cases/year in the district}$$

If the district programme registers 100 new patients when 200 are expected, the programme coverage is only 50% for the year. This indicates that the local health services need to question the effectiveness of the local TB control programme. This shows why it can be misleading to rely only on incidence or prevalence rates calculated from cases reported by the district's routine information system.

4.6 Seasonality

It is important to consider **seasonality** because morbidity and mortality patterns change with seasons and so do people's health responses and demands. In addition, services and programmes may be less well-organized during rainy and hot seasons. People's health-seeking behaviours can also show considerable seasonal variation. Analysis of health information by month and season is important for both health planning and management.

Seasons also affect households and their agricultural and employment activities. Seasons can affect subsistence farmers and poor urban workers through the availability of their food supplies and employment. For instance, malnutrition may be more common just before the harvest season and anopheline mosquitos increase with the onset of the rains. In West Africa, meningococcal meningitis epidemics increase with the onset of the dry *harmattan* wind season and end when the rains begin. In addition, road transport is often more difficult during the rains and people may use the health services less often. Supervision of health workers and health facilities may also be more difficult and essential drugs supplies may become unreliable.

4.7 Burden of disease

Health data can also be expressed as a composite indicator such as DALYs or HeaLYs that show disease burdens as a composite indicator that combines data on frequency, disability, morbidity and mortality (see Box 4.1).

These composite indicators are usually only valid for large national or re-gional populations and are not reliable for smaller district populations. However, they can assist in national decision by helping to identify priorities for health planning and resource allocation. For most purposes, however, using separate morbidity and mortality statistics is more useful in districts.

4.8 Health equity and inequalities

Epidemiology is concerned with the whole district population and local pla-nning needs to be both fair and impartial for everyone. For instance, achieving equity in access to health services and public health programmes is a priority regardless of people's social, ethnic, or cultural status but this requires that infor-mation is analysed for health inequalities at both district and national levels. This is done for inequalities when indicators are analysed with data based on sex, age, residence, ethnicity, education, socio-economic position, and migration.

District routine information systems can also provide data for estimates of age- and sex-specific incidence and prevalence and mortality rates which can help to understand how health problems or diseases are affecting different population subgroups. Routine systems often also provide information on

---

Box 4.1 Burden of disease in Pakistan, 1990

In Pakistan (population 112 million in 1990), a study using nearly 200 data sources estimated the burden of disease attributable to common conditions and calculated the loss of healthy life.

Overall 456 discounted HeaLYs per 1,000 people were lost due to new cases of diseases in 1990, 63% were through premature mortality, and 37% through disability. Loss of healthy life in Pakistan was less than that for countries in Sub-Saharan Africa but more than those in Latin America.

Diarrhoea and pneumonia in children caused the greatest loss of healthy life. Hypertension and injuries were the leading causes of healthy life lost from disability. Nearly half the healthy life lost occurred in the 0–4 years age group, showing the great burden among young children.

The review highlighted the importance of communicable diseases in Pakistan as causes of death, even though non-communicable diseases were the main cause of disability. Injuries were also a major public health problem.

Source data from Hyder 1998, and Hyder and Morrow 1999

residence which enables planners to compare indicator levels on people living in urban, peri-urban, rural, and isolated areas. Comparisons between different areas within districts is important.

Data collected by existing information systems need to gather information on inequalities. Ethnicity is particularly important in many multi-ethnic societies where some groups may have poor health indicators by being disadvantaged. However, recording ethnicity can be controversial and raise questions about whether this can unfairly discriminate against some minority groups. It also raises questions as how best to collect this data. In Brazil, for example, skin colour is required on all health forms, including on birth and death certificates, hospital admissions, and in surveillance systems.

Socio-economic data on education, income, occupation, and wealth are important but can be difficult to collect, although some information can be obtained using qualitative methods and using a range of questions (see Chapter 7) and by surveys (see Chapter 8). For example, maternal education is required in birth registration forms in Brazil. However, respondents may be reluctant to give truthful responses for some private information. At a minimum, it is important to disaggregate socio-economic indicators by age, sex, and area. Findings on inequalities should be routinely included in all health reports. For instance, education or schooling can be by level achieved, household income by wages, occupation by current and previous work, and wealth by ownership of different personal and household assets.

4.9 Health information checklist

Review of the collection and analysis of basic data:

- Symptoms and diseases included
- Diagnostic criteria used
- Facilities providing reports
- Reporting frequency and regularity
- Efforts made to regularly analyse data

Distribution and use of information:

- Use made by local health management team
- Distribution of information within district

- Feedback to local health facilities
- Reporting to regional and central authorities

Improving the routine information system:

- Correct common and obvious faults
- Effectiveness of reporting for important items
- Effects of seasonality
- Standardization of procedures
- In-service training for primary health care workers

Presentation of epidemiological information

- Most common diseases seen in out-patients and in-patients
- Most common causes of deaths in hospitals
- Distribution of common and epidemic diseases throughout district
- Inequalities by age, sex, and area for different socio-economic groups
- Other health problems

Frequency, distribution, and importance of health problems:

- Obstetric and gynaecological problems—prolonged labour, haemorrhage, retained placenta, puerperal fever, respiration and feeding in newborns, neonatal tetanus
- Common disorders—pneumonia, diarrhoea, malaria, malnutrition, measles, TB
- Endemic diseases—filariasis, HIV/AIDS, schistosomiasis, sexually transmitted infections, tetanus
- Potential epidemic diseases—pertussis, cholera, Ebola, meningitis, dengue, plague, typhoid, Covid-19
- Non-communicable diseases—accidents and injuries, hypertension, mental illness, anaemia

5

Reporting and Surveillance Systems

5.1 Routine health information

Each country will have its own **routine health information system** for collecting and reporting data from the periphery to the centre. Local health staff should be familiar with this system and appreciate what is required to make it work well. Figure 5.1 outlines such a system. Information is collected when people visit health services and programmes and data are written down and recorded. Later the information is analysed and communicated to health workers and to other local organizations. The Ministry of Health (MOH) or national statistics bureau is often responsible for collating this information for the whole country.

At the local level, the emphasis should be on collecting the minimum data in the simplest possible way. Data collected by health workers should be useful to them as well as their supervisors, and the local health team is in the best position to make good use of this principle.

Health information systems in many countries are often characterized by elaborate forms filled out in crowded outpatient clinics and hospitals and then sent for analysis centrally. This analysis can be delayed by months or even years and little feedback is passed to those collecting the original data. In addition, local health staff may have little or no input on the number or format of the forms used and have little influence on how well they are designed. Timely communication of the information is essential.

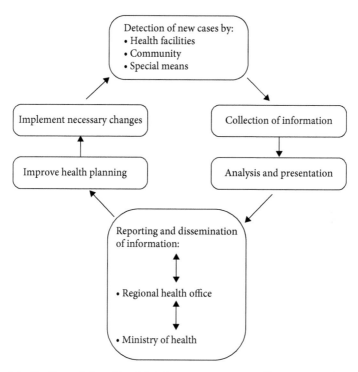

Figure 5.1 Outline of a local health information or surveillance system

Reproduced with permission from Vaughan, J Patrick, Morrow, Richard H, and World Health Organization, Manual of epidemiology for district health management, World Health Organization; Geneva, Switzerland, Copyright © 1989

Controlling the quality of data is vital and so are checks to ensure compliance with recommended procedures. Forms and procedures should be designed and tested to see if they are directly useful to both health workers themselves and their supervisors involved in local health services and programmes. National **reporting and surveillance** systems rely mainly on both the quantity and quality of this locally collected data.

Local data do not have to be complete to be useful. If the proportion of all cases detected remains reasonably constant over time the trends can be forecast, provided the problems and defects in data collection are well understood. This is illustrated by the number of poliomyelitis cases detected before and after the onset of a mass polio immunization campaign in Brazil (see Figure 5.2).

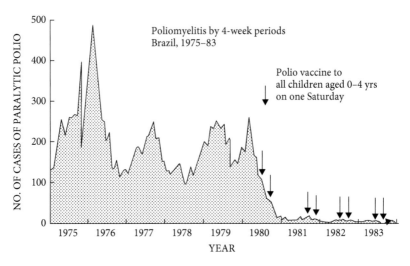

Figure 5.2 Incidence of poliomyelitis following a mass immunization campaign in Brazil

Reproduced with permission from Vaughan, J Patrick, Morrow, Richard H, and World Health Organization, Manual of epidemiology for district health management, World Health Organization; Geneva, Switzerland, Copyright © 1989

Even though all cases were probably not detected, the trend shows strong evidence that the incidence of polio was greatly reduced by the immunization campaigns.

5.2 Surveillance systems

Surveillance is the collection and analysis of incidence data and distribution as information on cases to answer the questions about who, where, and when. The term 'surveillance' can be used in different ways. In disease control and prevention programmes it involves collecting specific data on the factors that determine health risk behaviours and the incidence and distribution of cases. For global surveillance, World Health Organization (WHO) Member States are required to support the **International Health Regulations**, and some communicable diseases can be subject to international reporting. Surveillance can also refer to special reporting systems set up for particularly important health problems or diseases, including the spread of communicable diseases such as Covid-19, morbidity in natural disasters, or nutritional status in a famine. This kind of surveillance is usually organized for a limited time and is well integrated with the use of health interventions, such as the control of epidemic diseases like SARS or Ebola (see Box 5.1).

Box 5.1 Surveillance of Severe Acute Respiratory Syndrome (SARS)

The first known cases of SARS occurred in China in 2002 and this was followed by another major epidemic in 2003 that spread to 26 countries. It was believed that the SARS coronavirus (SARSCoV) was an animal virus that had crossed the species barrier due to increased human exposure to the virus.

The WHO developed a system for global surveillance and risk assessment while national governments retained responsibility for reporting. High-risk situations for the emergence of SARS were:

- Areas identified as source(s) of the epidemic in 2002–2003 in southern China which had an increased likelihood of animal-to-human transmission from wildlife or other animal reservoirs
- Presence of laboratories in which SARSCoV and/or SARSCoV-like viruses were being studied or in which infected and clinical specimens were being processed or stored
- Movement of large numbers of persons coming from areas with potential wildlife or other animal reservoirs of SARSCoV-like viruses

The SARS Covid-19 pandemic started in China in late 2019 and spread rapidly to many other countries, mainly through international travel. Early in 2020, the WHO emphasized the importance of testing for people infected with the virus and the role of tracing cases and isolation of contacts during the incubation period. In mid-2020, the WHO declared a global pandemic.

For more on SARS and Covid-19 see Section 6.9 and Section 6.10 for the Bangladesh case study, control measures Box 6.1, and ethics of freedom of movement Box 16.1.

Major uses of epidemiological surveillance include:

- Identifying outbreaks and epidemics and ensuring effective actions to control some diseases
- Monitoring implementation and effectiveness of intervention programmes by comparing the extent of the problem before and after the start of implementation of control measures
- Assisting health planning by showing which health and disease problems have significant priority

- Identifying high-risk groups (e.g. by age and occupation), geographical areas where the problem is common, and variations over time in incidence (e.g. seasonal and year-to-year transmission)
- Increasing the understanding and knowledge of vectors, animal reservoirs, and the modes and dynamics of transmission of some communicable and epidemic diseases

Other events that can require surveillance are: demographic events, such as births, marriages and deaths; epidemic diseases, such as yellow fever, dengue, meningococcal meningitis, haemorrhagic fever; behavioural health risks, such as unsafe sex, smoking, obesity, lack of physical exercise; nutritional status and malnutrition, including during famines, and for obesity; animal reservoirs and vectors for **zoonotic** communicable diseases such as plague; and environmental pollution for bacteria and chemicals, including for air and water pollution.

5.3 Definition of cases

Surveillance criteria for reporting **possible, probable, and definite** cases must be clear, realistic, and easy to understand. For example, the case definition used for surveillance of probable cholera may not include diarrhoea in children under five years old because this would increase the number of doubtful cases, while in surveillance for treatment of diarrhoea the cases could include all ages.

Health workers need training to use such case criteria correctly. This can be tested by giving staff short case descriptions and asking them to discuss how they would classify the cases and whether it should be reported. This helps to raise awareness among staff and to clarify any issues.

> DEFINE CRITERIA FOR REPORTING CASES AND TRAIN
> HEALTH WORKERS

Reported information should include the diagnosis and the frequency of cases, date of onset, illness duration, treatment, and whether the patient recovered or died. Also record patients' names, ages, sex, address, name of urban area or village, occupation, immunization or treatment status (if applicable). To enable follow-up of cases also include geographical location coordinates, place of infection and possible source, and neighbours for contact tracing. Urgent reporting is needed for potentially epidemic diseases. Information can be sent by mobile phone or e-mail message.

5.4 Sources of health information

The main sources of routinely reported information are:

- Health facilities
- Special searches
- Death certificates
- Laboratories
- Community surveillance
- Outbreak investigations
- Surveys and special studies

Health facility reports: The district office usually receives regular reports from all local health facilities, including hospitals, health centres, sub-centres, and mobile clinics, and also may be from private practitioners and community health workers. Reports can include cases and admissions by age, sex, diagnosis, and outcome. It is best for new out-patient visits to be recorded separately from repeat visits by age, sex, and diagnosis. For instance, this is best practice for antenatal visits, deliveries, family planning, child health, and attendances for sexually transmitted infections (STIs), tuberculosis, and other infectious diseases (see Table 5.1).

Vital registration: Reporting of births and deaths may not be the direct responsibility of the MOH nor the local team, but this information can be essential for local planning and management (see Chapter 3).

Laboratories: These provide information on confirmed diagnoses, especially of infectious diseases.

Table 5.1 Outline for reporting cases from a community health facility

Monthly report of new cases					
Health facility _____			Month ____		Year _____
Diagnosis	Name	Village	Age	Sex	Date of onset
1.					
2.					
3.					
4.					
Submitted by _____			Date __/__/__		

Special searches: These may involve schools, markets, particular villages, and high-risk households, and can be done by health workers or trained people such as teachers. Showing a picture of people with the disease and symptoms and signs may be helpful. The person's address, name, age, and sex, and household mobile photograph can be used for later follow-up, particularly in outbreaks when active case finding is essential (see Chapter 6).

Surveys and special studies: These can be useful for the periodic surveillance of some conditions. There can be, however, both over-reporting and under-reporting of cases which can be difficult to detect and correct. It is helpful to compare the incidence in previous years for the same time period.

Community surveillance: Many diseases are well recognized by local people who give them local names, and are easily recognized by community health workers, traditional birth attendants, and community groups who can inform primary-level health facilities (see Figure 5.3). This kind of surveillance

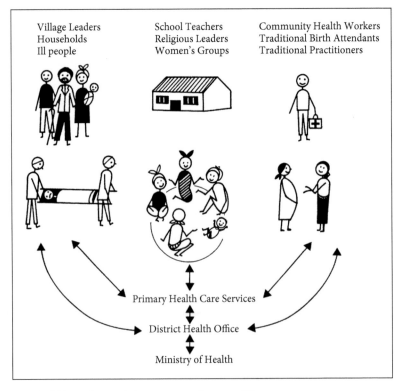

Figure 5.3 Ways of organizing community surveillance

Reproduced with permission from Vaughan, J Patrick, Morrow, Richard H, and World Health Organization, Manual of epidemiology for district health management, World Health Organization; Geneva, Switzerland, Copyright © 1989

may be useful in special programmes, such as for malaria control and family planning. Schoolteachers, religious leaders, and government administrative officers can be helpful in reporting cases, and so can local radio and television, both of which can be helpful for publicity, especially in more remote areas.

5.5 Analysis and presentation of data

Collected data must be analysed and presented simply. How this is done will depend on the local information system and the following is only a guide. A register is a book or file containing the recorded data for all similar cases or diagnoses with all data entered into one register as part of the local information system.

Cases should be reported by date of onset, but in practice they are often reported by date of first attendance and/or diagnosis. Tables can be prepared for:

- *Who?* (e.g. age and sex, Table 5.2)
- *Where?* (e.g. village of onset, Table 5.3)
- *When?* (e.g. cases per day, week or month, see Figure 5.4)

Incidence by month can be very variable with seasonal changes, such as for new cholera cases in Figure 5.4. This shows that in practice, total cases can be more useful than calculating a rate. However, to compare incidence between different districts or population groups and between different time periods it is best to calculate age- and sex-specific rates or to use standardized rates (see Annex One).

ANALYSE ALL CASES ACCORDING TO WHO? WHERE? WHEN?

Table 5.2 Suggested table for analysis of cases by age and sex

Disease or health problem					Reporting period	
Sex	Age group (years)					
	0–4	5–14	15–44	45–64	65+	Total
Male						
Female						
Total						

Table 5.3 Suggested table for analysis of cases by place of onset

Disease or health problem					Reporting period
Number of cases by place (e.g. village)					
A	B	C	D	E	Total

5.6 Using data and information

Reporting surveillance data should help to improve the management of local services. If reported data and information are not used, a reporting or surveillance system can be a waste of time and money!

Reported information must be communicated to all relevant authorities, including:

- Primary health care workers involved in sending in the original data and reports

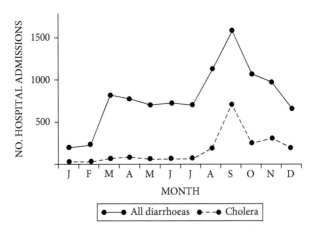

Figure 5.4 Seasonality of hospital admissions for all diarrhoea and cholera cases by month

Reproduced with permission from Vaughan, J Patrick, Morrow, Richard H, and World Health Organization, Manual of epidemiology for district health management, World Health Organization; Geneva, Switzerland, Copyright © 1989

- Health facility and district staff, community health teams and local health committees
- Regional and national staff, so they can compile information for many different areas
- Workers involved in organizing community health programmes
- Village councils and other local organizations
- Non-governmental, voluntary, and private health services
- Local social media, local radio stations, and newspapers

> **WILL THE INFORMATION BE USED? WHAT DIFFERENCE WILL IT MAKE?**

5.7 Reporting systems checklist

Diseases or health problems being reported:

- Reporting of cases, episodes, or attendances?
- Diagnostic criteria and working definitions being used
- Estimates of any possible under- and over-reporting

Sources of health information:

- Health facilities
- Vital registration (births and deaths)
- Laboratories
- Community leaders
- Special searches
- Outbreak investigations
- Health surveys and studies

Analysis and presentation:

- Registers
- Files
- Monthly graphs
- Spot maps
- Special reports

Communicate findings to:

- MOH and regions
- Primary health care workers and district staff
- Village councils and organizations
- Non-governmental, voluntary, and private health organizations
- Local social and mass media, radio

Using information in health planning:

- Coverage of reporting and surveillance system
- Improvements to community health programmes
- Improvements in district health plans
- Use of information in community health education
- Changes in district health status indicators

6

Outbreaks and Epidemics

6.1 Communicable diseases

Communicable diseases are often the commonest cause of outpatient clinical attendances and hospital admissions, although the pattern can vary considerably during different seasons and between different districts. These diseases are usually caused by an infection that is a living **agent**, such as a virus (e.g. Covid-19, Zika, influenza), bacteria (e.g. shigella dysentery, meningococcal meningitis), or protozoa (e.g. malaria, trypanosomiasis).

Some of these diseases can spread or be propagated directly from one person to another human host. To control **chains of transmission** epidemiology considers the relationships between the **agent, host**—people or an animal—and the **environment** in which they live. People are the main host for most human infectious diseases and some are zoonotic from other animals.

Infections can result from **exposure** to the **source** of the agent which can then lead to onward transmission (see Figure 6.1). Transmission can be by:

- Direct and close contact, e.g. Ebola, human immunodeficiency virus (HIV), leprosy

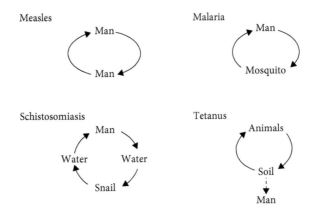

Figure 6.1 Source and transmission of some communicable diseases

- Airborne droplets, e.g. Covid-19, measles, tuberculosis (TB)
- Contamination of food, water, or soil, e.g. amoebic dysentery, food poisoning, tetanus
- Vectorborne, e.g. malaria, schistosomiasis, leishmaniasis
- Contact with infected animals, e.g. rabies, plague

For transmission to occur the new host must be both **exposed** to the agent and **susceptible** to being infected. Transmission also depends on the dose of the organisms during exposure; the higher the dose the more likely that this will lead to infection. Exposure can result in no transmission at all, or a subclinical infection which can be difficult to detect and diagnose, or a more serious and clinical infection with symptoms and signs.

A **susceptible** host is one that lacks immunity or has only a partial resistance to an infectious agent causing the communicable disease. Susceptibility to the agent and little or weak resistance can be due to:

- Exposure of the population to a totally new agent, e.g. Covid-19
- Immunity not yet acquired to the agent, e.g. measles in infants
- Weak protective immunity, e.g. malaria
- Severe illness, e.g. TB and HIV
- Malnutrition, e.g. diarrhoea, respiratory infections
- Immuno-suppression, e.g. chemotherapy, cancers

Control of most communicable diseases relies on lowering the chain of transmission and the number of new cases by reducing exposure to the source of the agent, interrupting the mode of transmission, and by protecting susceptible hosts. This is explained further in Section 6.6.

6.2 Definition of an outbreak or epidemic

A local disease outbreak or small **epidemic** is commonly defined as the occurrence in a community or area of cases clearly in excess of what is expected. An outbreak or epidemic may be confirmed by comparing the incidence of disease cases with that in previous years for a similar period in the same community.

The term 'epidemic' is relative to the previous incidence of the disease in the same area, among specified population groups, and at different seasons of the year. The appearance of two cases of plague may constitute an outbreak whereas a high incidence of diarrhoeal diseases during the peak season may be considered 'normal'. In addition, some diseases can show marked seasonal and annual variations in incidence, such as measles and meningococcal meningitis.

Epidemics happen in different ways in different communities, but health workers still need to follow a systematic approach both to investigating them and for the epidemic control measures, as shown in Figure 6.2. Both should be undertaken at the same time.

Local outbreaks and epidemics are most often due to communicable diseases with a short **incubation period** and which are easily transmitted,

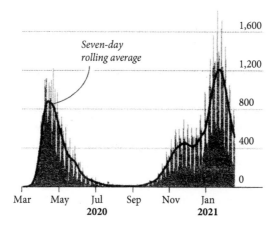

Figure 6.2 Seven day rolling average for new Covid-19 deaths, United Kingdom 2020–2021

Source data from data.gov.uk

such as food-borne shigella and water-borne cholera. Whether an epidemic exists or not can be a highly political issue and it is advisable for health workers to seek help from their senior colleagues before making any public announcements.

Transmission can also involve **disease vectors** as in malaria, **intermediate hosts** such as snails in schistosomiasis, and a **zoonosis** when the infection is transmitted from other animals such as for yellow fever and plague.

Local outbreaks are commonly due to:

- Foodborne outbreaks, e.g. *Escherichia coli*, shigella, staphylococcal infection, salmonellosis
- Communicable diseases with short incubation periods, e.g. Covid, dengue, cholera, Ebola, influenza, malaria, measles, plague, typhoid, typhus, yellow fever
- Communicable diseases with longer incubation periods, e.g. HIV/ acquired immunodeficiency syndrome (AIDS), African trypanosomiasis, viral hepatitis, kala-azar
- Toxic substances, e.g. contaminated foods, insecticides, agricultural chemicals

6.3 Serious epidemics and pandemics

Epidemics due to severe acute respiratory syndrome (SARS), Covid-19, and Ebola are uncommon and Ministries of Health (MOH) may only experience a major epidemic every few years. **Pandemics** occurs when epidemic transmission spreads to many countries, and a global pandemic, such as Covid-19, is when the disease spreads rapidly and many cases occur in most countries and continents. Before Covid-19, the last global pandemic was the H1N1 avian influenza outbreak in 2009. The 1918 Spanish influenza pandemic caused an estimated 50 million deaths worldwide and is believed to have been caused by an H1N1 virus of avian origin.

Severe acute respiratory syndrome (SARS) and Covid-19 are examples of aerosol and droplet infection leading to **person-to-person or propagated transmission** and a rapid outbreak will occur if a high proportion of people are both susceptible and exposed and do not have any immunity to the agent causing the epidemic. Some highly infectious diseases, such as the Covid-19 virus, may also cause asymptomatic, sub-clinical, or mild illnesses with few symptoms or signs that can be difficult to detect without a specific viral test. Asymptomatic and mildly infected cases may still be able to transmit the virus to other susceptible people, with such transmission only being detected with specific virus or antibody laboratory tests.

If Covid-19 transmission causes one case to lead to an average of more than one newly infected case, the incidence will increase and an epidemic can eventually occur. If one case leads on average of two or more new cases, an epidemic will occur very rapidly over a short time period and the agent will quickly spread in the wider population. Figure 6.2 shows that in the United Kingdom from October 2020 to early February 2021, the epidemic went from a few deaths per day to about 1,200 per day. This was due to the **reproduction rate R** being much higher than 1.0 particularly in the elderly and vulnerable population. A seven-day rolling average is used to smooth out variations in the daily deaths.

Deaths in the United Kingdom decreased when national lockdown measures were enforced and the transmission rate R then began to fall. The aim of controlling of a propagated epidemic is to lower the transmission and sustain the R value at less than an average of one when this kind of epidemic should slow down and stop due to a fall in the number of new infections. Since the R value is an average across the population, transmission can at the same time be higher in some areas and lower in others.

The main steps in the investigation and control of a local outbreak or epidemic are shown in Figure 6.3. This starts with a review of all the reported **cases** to analyse the clinical case histories and the need for any **laboratory tests** to confirm the diagnosis. It is most important that control measures are started as soon as possible.

Corona viruses like Covid-19 commonly mutate their genetic structure and develop new **variants** which can be more infectious. This can lead to an increase in transmission and a higher R rate and hence a rapidly expanding epidemic. A major concern is whether these variants also become more virulent and reduce the efficacy of new vaccines and thus make it harder to bring the Covid-19 epidemic under control. Early in 2021, new variants were reported in the United Kingdom, Brazil, South Africa, and a number of other countries.

6.4 Confirming an outbreak or epidemic

Urgent action may be based on the clinical diagnosis alone before waiting for results and before consulting more experienced public health specialists.

> **USE DIAGNOSTIC CRITERIA FOR POSSIBLE, PROBABLE, AND DEFINITE CASES**

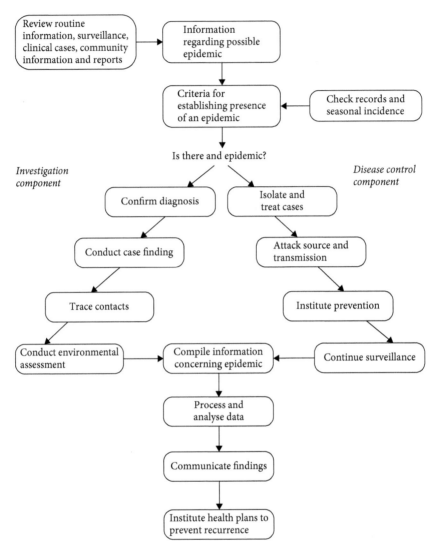

Figure 6.3 Outline of the investigation and control of a possible epidemic

Reproduced with permission from Vaughan, J Patrick, Morrow, Richard H, and World Health Organization, Manual of epidemiology for district health management, World Health Organization; Geneva, Switzerland, Copyright © 1989

It is important to recognize a potential epidemic early and to understand its possible cause and method of transmission. Control measures should then start as soon as possible. An outbreak or local epidemic may be reported first by community members and leaders like teachers, police, and health workers. Outbreaks may also be detected when ill patients report to health centres and unexpected deaths occur in hospitals. These should be recorded by the local health information and surveillance system.

It is important to immediately establish diagnostic criteria for **possible, probable, and definite cases,** particularly when new cases cannot easily be diagnosed clinically and when the disease may be spreading through **subclinical** or **asymptomatic** infections.

An epidemic or outbreak is most likely to be explained by analysing the definite cases. It is also important to use clear criteria when searching for other possible cases and when using **contact tracing** to follow up for other possible cases. Criteria for cases may need to be modified later as more is understood about the cause of the epidemic and its transmission.

Initial interviews with cases need to record case histories with the variety of symptoms and clinical signs and possible explanations for the outbreak included, and these histories can be developed at this early stage. In epidemics, health workers need to encourage and reinforce public trust, particularly when people are asked to give confidential details of their illness and asked for their possible contacts when identifying other potential cases.

A **cluster epidemic** is when many susceptible people are simultaneously exposed and infected by a common source. For yellow fever and cholera only a few cases may need to be investigated to confirm the epidemic. However, it is important when investigating an outbreak to remember that some cases may be sub-clinical or mild and only identified by detailed inquiries or specific laboratory tests.

PREVENT TRANSMISSION BY TESTING, TRACING, AND ISOLATING CASES

Case detection can also involve undertaking special searches to find any additional unreported or unsuspected cases. This is especially true for some chronic diseases such as HIV/AIDS, where testing and antenatal screening can provide useful contact information for other people with possible disease.

When the outbreak **source** is known, further cases may be identified through contact tracing and by testing other people exposed to the same possible source. This is essential when cases must be treated or isolated to prevent further spread. Contact tracing is easiest for disease of short duration and can be more difficult for illnesses with long incubation periods and for asymptomatic and sub-clinical infections.

6.5 Describing the outbreak or epidemic

It is important to analyse the cases by the categories of who, where, and when in order to identify any common characteristics. Are there any similarities between the cases? Descriptive epidemiology collects information on all known cases for such variables as age, sex, residence, and occupation, as well as for possible dates of exposure and time of onset during the possible incubation period. Initially the actual numbers of cases may be used but later age- and sex-specific **attack rates** may be needed. **Incubation periods** are best expressed as the median and range in days. Long incubation periods, such as for HIV/AIDS, mean the cases will be more spread out over a longer period of time.

WHAT DO ALL KNOWN CASES HAVE IN COMMON?

Basic questions about an outbreak or epidemic are:

- What is the organism or agent or chemical causing the outbreak?
- What is the source of exposure?
- What is the possible mode of exposure and transmission?
- How can the epidemic be explained?
- How can the epidemic be controlled?

Knowledge of possible **exposures** and routes for chains of transmission can help to focus the investigation. For example, in cases with fever malaria is usually transmitted by night-biting mosquitoes (*Anopheles*) so it is important to find out where people sleep, whereas dengue fever is transmitted by day-biting mosquitoes (*Aedes*) mosquitoes and daily activities and work routines may be important. Chemical exposures may be due to occupations such as farming and manufacturing.

POINT-SOURCE EPIDEMICS HAVE CASES WITHIN ONE INCUBATION PERIOD

Epidemic incidence curve (when?)

This is a graph that plots cases of the disease against time of onset which may indicate the nature of the outbreak and the possible source. A **point-source outbreak** is one with a common exposure of susceptible people to a pathogen

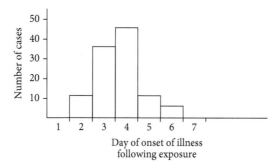

Figure 6.4 Epidemic curve of a point-source outbreak

Reproduced with permission from Vaughan, J Patrick, Morrow, Richard H, and World Health Organization, Manual of epidemiology for district health management, World Health Organization; Geneva, Switzerland, Copyright © 1989

or agent at one point in time. New cases then occur over a short time period that is similar to the **incubation period** of the disease. Figure 6.4 shows a typical epidemic curve. Exposure is assumed to have taken place on day zero and the incubation period appears to be two to six days with an average of four days. This is similar to that expected for a point source epidemic such as cholera outbreak and food-borne diseases.

Person-to-person transmission can lead onto a **propagated epidemic**, such as can occur in shigellosis, influenza, or Covid-19 virus. In Figure 6.5 the source case is unknown and the first detected cases appeared on the 13th day of the month, with subsequent cases appearing at about 3-day intervals. The R value will be greater than one and the shape of the epidemic curve depends on the incubation period of the disease and whether the environment favours transmission.

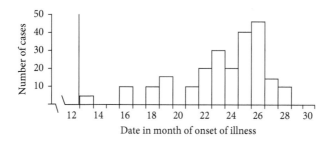

Figure 6.5 Epidemic curve for a propagated epidemic

Reproduced with permission from Vaughan, J Patrick, Morrow, Richard H, and World Health Organization, Manual of epidemiology for district health management, World Health Organization; Geneva, Switzerland, Copyright © 1989

Person-to-person transmission can also lead to an extended point-source outbreak due to the continuous exposure and transmission occurring over a longer period of time. There is often an abrupt onset but new cases will be spread over a period longer than the possible incubation period.

An epidemic curve can provide the probable time of exposure and may indicate the organism or agent and its incubation period. For example, if Figure 6.3 represents a cholera outbreak, then exposure seems to have occurred 2 to 5 days (the usual incubation period for cholera) before days 3 and 4 when most cases occurred. Similarly, if the epidemic in Figure 6.5 was a shigellosis outbreak and the first case recognized on day 3 and exposure to a possible source case was about 3 days earlier, the incubation period for shigellosis. This can help trace the source of the infection, such as contaminated or infected food. Conversely, if the date/time of exposure is known, the incubation period can be calculated, which can give a clue to the cause. This often applies in foodborne disease outbreaks when the time of exposure is often known. For example, if the epidemic in Figure 6.4 was a food poisoning outbreak and the meal had been taken at midday on day 2, the median incubation period could be calculated as about 24 hours, which suggests salmonella or staphylococcus food poisoning.

In outbreaks due to person-to-person spread the degree of crowding and intimacy of contact, for instance within households, will determine the speed at which the epidemic reaches a peak, while the proportion of the population that is susceptible will influence the extent of the outbreak. For vector-borne diseases the agent develops in the vector and conditions that favour the vector can also affect the epidemic curve.

6.6 Analysis of cases by who, where, when

Descriptive analysis according to who, where, and when may be sufficient to indicate the source of an outbreak, the agent, chain of transmission, and the appropriate control measures. Marking known cases on a **spot map** (see Figure 6.6) may indicate a possible source but it is also important to consider the distribution of the general population. For example, if 70% of the population live in the local town, why are most cases coming from rural areas?

For other outbreaks further analysis may be necessary, such as cases according to age, sex, and occupation, which may give clues to the source. Cases in children may suggest a source in their homes or at school, whereas if adult

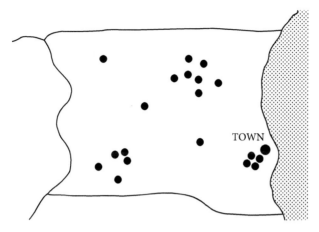

Figure 6.6 District spot map showing clusters of epidemic cases

Reproduced with permission from Vaughan, J Patrick, Morrow, Richard H, and World Health Organization, Manual of epidemiology for district health management, World Health Organization; Geneva, Switzerland, Copyright © 1989

males are mainly affected the source may be at work or among social contacts. Attack rates can be useful to compare exposure in different groups.

When cases of diarrhoea occur within a short time period (e.g. over about two to three days for shigellosis, four to six days for cholera, and two weeks for typhoid) are marked on the spot map in one colour and subsequent cases in another colour, the epidemic pattern can quickly become apparent. Clustering of cases in one area at about the same time, called **space-time clustering**, indicates the possibility of a localized epidemic due to a point-source exposure.

6.7 Case-control analysis

In a **case-control** analysis the cases are asked questions on their activities to see what possible exposures they have in common within the possible incubation period, such as to foods, drinking water, work, or sexual behaviours. The same questions are also asked of a control group of people living in the same area who do not have the disease. These people should be of the same sex and age (within five years). It is preferable to have two control persons for every known case who live in neighbouring households but who are well. Recalling activities can be difficult and the same checklist must be used for both cases and controls. It is important to avoid asking leading questions. The data from cases

Table 6.1 Case-control study of 18 cholera cases according to water source used

	Water source used			
	TOTAL	A	B	C
Cases	18	17	16	6
Controls	18	14	3	17
TOTAL	36	31	19	23

and controls are then analysed for any significant differences between the two groups for exposure to all possible sources.

Table 6.1 is an example where three sources of drinking water were suspected in a cholera outbreak. To determine the true origin of the infection, the cases and controls were all questioned about their sources of drinking water in the previous two to three days before the onset of the outbreak. Water source B appears to be the most likely cause, even though each person probably had used more than one source of water. The longer the incubation period the more difficult it is to use this technique.

If only the 18 cases had been questioned the likely source could have been either A (17) or B (16). However, the controls in B had drunk less and therefore B is the most likely source. The difference between the cases and controls is important and statistical testing may sometimes be necessary.

What about the two cases who had apparently not taken water from source B (total 18, B 16)? People are often unaware of their water source or they could have used water from several sources. People can also give wrong answers. The three controls who said they had water from B may not in fact have done so or they just did not become infected or develop the disease.

Another useful method, particularly for food-borne epidemics, is to compare attack rates among those having eaten particular foods when rates will be higher than among the unexposed.

6.8 Controlling outbreaks or epidemics

Steps for investigating and controlling an epidemic are outlined in Figures 6.3 above and the main methods for controlling communicable diseases are summarized in Table 6.2 below.

Table 6.2 Summary of strategies to control an epidemic due to a communicable disease

Attack the source	Interrupt transmission	Protecting susceptibles
Identify cases	Personal hygiene	Immunization
Treat cases and carriers	Environmental hygiene	Chemoprophylaxis
Isolate cases and suspects	Vector control	Personal protection
Trace all contacts	Universal precautions	Better nutrition
Control animal reservoirs	Disinfection/sterilization	Health education
Notify cases	Stop people movements	Behaviour modification
Educate population	Start safe social distancing	Start safe distancing

Laboratory examination of suspected food or water for toxic chemicals or faecal contamination may indicate an environmental source for the outbreak. In vector-borne diseases it may be necessary to investigate possible vector-breeding sites.

When the causative organism or agent, its source, and the exposure and route of transmission are known it will probably be possible to explain why the epidemic occurred. Control measures depend on identifying the actual disease concerned.

Primary prevention is about preventing new cases and this is achieved mainly by the measures listed under 'interrupt transmission' and under 'protecting susceptibles', together with contact tracing, and control of vectors or animal reservoirs. If these measures are implemented well and quickly in a propagated epidemic, the R-reproductive rate should fall to below 1 when new cases will be reduced over time and the outbreak will stop.

Clean water supplies and the correct disposal of faeces will prevent the spread of cholera, control of anopheline mosquitoes will reduce malaria transmission, immunization protects young children against measles, and condoms and modification of sexual behaviours should reduce the number of individuals newly infected with HIV.

Vaccines can be very effective in protecting susceptible individuals provided they have a high efficacy and the population immunization coverage is also high. A commonly accepted efficacy for a vaccine is that it should provide 80% protection or more in susceptible individuals. However, protection may be reduced if the virus or agent develops strains that are resistant to the vaccine and unfortunately many viruses can mutate, which can lead to vaccines becoming less effective.

Secondary and tertiary prevention can stop the spread from established cases and is achieved by finding sub-clinical cases and carriers, by contact tracing and surveillance. Tertiary prevention relies on treating cases, carriers, and animal reservoirs so they do not spread the organism or agent any further.

In outbreaks due to person-to-person transmission, control can involve stopping population movements in and out of the affected area, isolation of all known and quarantining of possible cases, and installing safe social distancing between people particularly in confined areas such as in households and in public areas.

Attacking the source and mode of transmission may involve cleaning contaminated water sources and restricting access to them, destroying infected food, eliminating or spraying vector-breeding sites, and preventing further use of dangerous chemicals.

In epidemics, maintaining public trust is crucial, and health education and mass media communications are very important for public support in limiting the source and mode of transmission. Public guidelines and legislation may also be necessary. Control measures can include:

- Testing for possible cases and tracing all contacts
- Treating and isolating cases and quarantining possible cases. Total isolation may be necessary for highly infectious diseases as Ebola, haemorrhagic fevers, and Covid-19
- Increasing the resistance of the local population, for instance against malaria and meningococcal meningitis with chemoprophylaxis and with immunization for measles

In some epidemics, vaccination can lead people to have a false confidence that the epidemic is under control. After the acute phase it is usual to continue with surveillance for possible cases and suspects. Once the epidemic is under control, ongoing **surveillance** for new cases will show if the control measures have been effective. Routine reporting systems may not be adequate for this and special surveillance and community reporting may have to be organized.

6.9 Covid-19 and previous SARS epidemics

The SARS first epidemic occurred in China in 2002 and this was followed by another major epidemic in 2003 that spread to 26 countries. It was believed that the SARS coronavirus (SARSCoV) was an animal virus that had crossed the species barrier due to increased human exposure to the virus. The World Health Organization (WHO) developed a system for surveillance and risk assessment with national governments taking responsibility for reporting all cases and deaths (see Box 5.1). The epidemic was eventually controlled by lowering the R-rate of transmission to less than 1 by strictly controlling population movements, isolating all known cases, widespread testing for new cases, social distancing, and closing down of public spaces.

The onset of the global Covid-19 pandemic, which also began in China in 2019, was also caused by a SARS-like virus which is highly infectious and easily transmitted between people by aerosol droplets due to coughing and sneezing, particularly when people are crowded together in enclosed indoor spaces like households, shops, and eating places. This virus probably also crossed over from an animal species.

Covid-19 is a completely new virus variant for human populations which means that people have no previous immunity and there is no apparent cross-over immunity from previous infections with other coronaviruses. The global pandemic is the result, therefore, of a new and highly infectious virus spreading rapidly in non-immune human populations. In addition, although many cases are asymptomatic or mild, and therefore difficult to detect, these can still be infectious and therefore transmit the virus to infect new susceptible people.

Effective vaccines against Covid-19 have been developed and by late 2020 had already been declared safe and effective by regulatory agencies in Europe and the United States. Some countries then began to roll out national vaccination programmes based mainly on first protecting the elderly, the most vulnerable and key workers, and then gradually immunizing other age groups.

The main control measures for Covid-19 are shown in Box 6.1 below.

However, despite the rapid increase in cases detected in such countries as the United Kingdom, the United States, Bangladesh, and Brazil, the population sero-positivity level for protective antibodies in late 2020 was probably still only around 10%. This means that about 90% of the population had not yet been infected nor vaccinated and therefore had not yet developed any possible immunity.

A commonly accepted efficacy for a new vaccine is that it should provide 80% protection or more in susceptible individuals and new vaccines against Covid-19 have been shown in controlled efficacy trials to be effective in protecting susceptible individuals. However, vaccines may not prevent onward transmission

---

Box 6.1 Main methods for controlling the transmission of Covid-19

Isolating cases and suspects: Cases may be identified by symptoms—such as fever, persistent cough, loss of taste and smell—and/or testing for the virus. Cases are usually isolated for two weeks

Contact tracing: identifying and monitoring people who may have come into contact with an infectious person. Monitoring Covid-19 usually involves quarantine to control any spread

Personal protective equipment (PPE): specialized equipment to protect health workers and vulnerable people against exposure to the virus by aerosols via the nose, mouth, eyes, and hands

Social distancing: separating people by maintaining physical distance to prevent transmission of Covid-19, including keeping at least two metres apart, remote working, and cancelling events

Lockdown: emergency measures to control exposure and transmission by restricting people's movements and travel and encouraging people to stay at home and to isolate themselves

Immunization: by late 2020, new vaccines had been developed and become available for mass vaccination campaigns, with priority given first to the elderly, vulnerable and health care workers

---

of the virus and the immune response may fade over time. Despite vaccines having a high efficacy controlling the epidemic requires that the population immunity due to infection or vaccination probably has to be about 70% or higher. To achieve this high level, large-scale vaccination programmes need to be rolled out, especially to protect the vulnerable, elderly, and health care and other key workers.

Like the influenza viruses, the SARS viruses can mutate, and new Covid-19 co-variants were detected in late 2020 in the United Kingdom, Brazil, South Africa, and other countries. During 2021 more variants were expected to appear in other countries and these can be spread through international travel. Some new variants are even more infectious and have raised the R-rate by about 30–50% which has led to the rapid onset of national epidemics, an expansion in the number of new cases and higher case mortality rates. New mutations may also alter the efficacy of vaccines, and the effectiveness of control measures may be reduced, making epidemics harder to control. As with influenza vaccines, in future it may be necessary to modify the Covid-19 vaccines if their efficacy and protection are reduced by the new variants.

6.10 Bangladesh case study of the Covid-19 epidemic

Bangladesh illustrates the rapid spread of SARS-CoV-2 (severe acute respiratory syndrome, coronavirus 2), known as the Covid-19 pandemic. It showed the typical pattern for the rapid onset of the Covid-19 epidemic—see Figure 6.7 which shows the 7 DMA (7-day moving average) for confirmed Covid-19 cases and deaths.

The first Bangladesh country cases were identified in March 2020 in migrants returning home from Italy. Bangladesh is a densely populated country with many people living in crowded slums and households, and who travel around in crowded buses, trains, and ferries. Covid-19 infection spread rapidly and quickly caused a countrywide epidemic. The first recorded deaths occurred in mid-March 2020 and a national lockdown was imposed for two months from late March to the end of May, although there was weak enforcement of social distancing and hygiene measures.

Early on, the capital city Dhaka and port city of Chattagram had the highest number of cases and deaths. This rapidly reached a peak for cases around

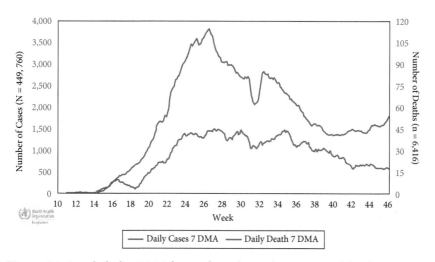

Figure 6.7 Bangladesh 7 DMA for confirmed Covid-19 cases and deaths
8 March–23 November 2020 Source: WHO (2020).

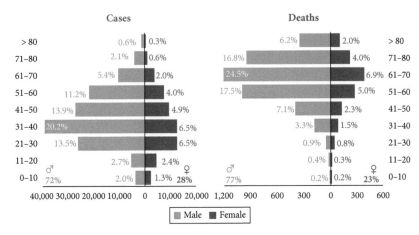

Figure 6.8 Bangladesh Covid-19 cases and deaths, 8 March–26 October 2020
Source: WHO (2020).

June and July 2020 when the virus had probably already spread throughout Bangladesh. Confirmed deaths continued throughout 2020 but rose more slowly about three weeks later and declined more slowly thereafter. Figure 6.8 shows that recorded cases were mainly among men in the mobile 20–60 years age range and reported deaths were mainly in men aged 50 years and older. However, it is difficult to estimate what proportion of all cases and deaths were actually tested and correctly reported.

An economic stimulus package of about 3% of gross domestic product (GDP) was started but less than 0.1% of this was allocated for health, the second lowest globally. There was considerable public concern about the rising epidemic and the government's apparent lack of a national control strategy. There were also calls for an urgent overhaul of the health system to improve primary health care and the stronger implementation of Universal Health Coverage (UHC). This was typical of the situation seen in many other countries.

For more on SARS and Covid-19 see Box 5.1 for surveillance, Section 6.9 for epidemiology, Box 6.1 for control measures, and Box 16.1 for ethics of controlling freedom of movement.

6.11   Reporting an outbreak or epidemic

The investigation and control of major epidemics is the responsibility of national MOH and the WHO collates the global information. For local outbreaks the district health authorities should report them as soon as possible to regional health authorities and the MOH. When the outbreak or epidemic is under control, a brief written report covering the following points should be circulated with recommendations for the control of any similar outbreaks in future:

- Causative organism or agent and probable sources and means of exposure and transmission
- Description of epidemic curve, geographical distribution, and main features of the cases
- Possible reason(s) for the outbreak or epidemic
- Disease control measures undertaken
- Recommendations for improvements to prevent recurrence of the epidemic

Copies of the report can be distributed to district government officers, health workers in charge of other district health facilities, non-government agencies, private health providers, community leaders, and other local organizations.

6.12 District epidemic checklist

Is there an outbreak or epidemic?

- review cases for possible diseases
- identify susceptibles and high-risk groups
- define diagnostic criteria for possible, probable, and definite cases
- check health information reporting for new cases
- search for other missed cases
- review previous incidence levels for endemicity and local knowledge

Describe the outbreak:

- who? characteristics of cases
- where? mapping of cases
- when? epidemic incidence curve
- collect information on populations at risk to establish denominators

What caused the outbreak?

- causative organism or agent
- exposure, source, and transmission

- case control method to test explanations
- send specimens for laboratory investigations

Institute control measures for the particular disease:

- control population movements in and out of the area
- introduce safe distancing measures
- test susceptibles
- trace and isolate contacts
- control the source and interrupt transmission
- protect susceptible people
- notify authorities

Write and distribute report.

- write and distribute report
- communicate findings
- make recommendations

DEFINE CASES AND THEN DETECT, TEST, TRACE, AND ISOLATE

7

Using Qualitative Methods

7.1 Using qualitative information

Qualitative methods can be quick and flexible and allow people to reveal their perceptions and beliefs about local health services safely. These methods can provide useful insights into the local context and reveal people's impressions and understanding on the delivery, access, quality, and coverage of local health services and programmes. These methods can also help support dialogue with community representatives. This all helps to understand issues such as perceptions about the quality of local health services, barriers to public use, reasons for low coverage, concerns about costs and fees, and different cultural beliefs and health-seeking behaviours.

It is important to use several different study approaches to see if they show similar findings and conclusions. Triangulation is when similar or the same findings come from different qualitative approaches. For example, why is coverage low for immunization and reproductive health services when vaccines and family planning are available at local health facilities? The advantages and disadvantages of these methods are summarized in Table 7.1.

```
QUALITATIVE METHODS GIVE INSIGHTS INTO PERCEPTIONS
AND BELIEFS
```

Table 7.1 Advantages and disadvantages of selected qualitative methods

Method	Advantages	Disadvantages
Record reviews	Useful information on patient illnesses and attendances Valuable insights into quality of services and provision of care	Subject to biases due to selective sample of attendances Inadequate case note information Poor diagnosis and weak case notes
Making observations	Records actual behaviours Can help rapport with community cooperation Implementation can be easy Can suggest causal links Some findings are quantifiable	Observed people may act adversely Can be time-consuming Observers need good training Some behaviours difficult to observe Can miss new or rare behaviours
Patient facility exit interviews	Quick comments on satisfaction Assesses quality of local services Checks on treatment provided Follow-up on advice provided	Patients using services are unlikely to say they are dissatisfied Answers can be biased if asked by health workers themselves
Indepth interviews	Interviews can cover wide topics Can put issues into local context Useful for local perceptions Data may be compared over time Use standard interviewer forms	Small number of informants Requires highly skilled interviewers Respondents unaware of issues Respondents may think they are being 'tested'
Focus groups	Provides information on opinions and insights Encourages debate on key topics Can identify public concerns	May not reveal sensitive behaviours May avoid sensitive local problems Logistical difficulties for meetings and groups
Participatory rural appraisal	Community creates the data map Encourages good rapport of people with investigators Can show seasonal variations	Sample may be unrepresentative Emphasis on public views only Sensitivities may be hidden

7.2 Record reviews

The analysis of recorded information and data, such as patient case notes, can provide useful management information about staff, patient attendances, available drug stocks, and variety of medicines dispensed. Reviews also provide simple but valuable insights into service quality. However, findings can be subject to biases due to the selected nature of the information and because of the inadequate and poor-quality case notes.

In-patient case reviews can be very helpful for identifying problems with the quality of clinical care, for example with obstetric care in Box 7.1.

Box 7.1 Review of obstetric care at a district hospital

A local health team identified that there was a serious problem of high maternal mortality with in-patient baby deliveries. A review of patient case records for hospital maternal deaths confirmed that sepsis, haemorrhage, obstructed labour, and hypertensive disease accounted for nearly all these deaths.

However, this review also found that nearly all mothers dying of sepsis had acquired their infection after admission to hospital. A thorough review of all the patient records for obstetric procedures indicated that staff needed further training, and deep cleaning of wards and operating theatres was also urgently required. These were carried out and this led quickly to fewer cases of sepsis and later, to a reduction in maternal mortality in the hospital. These improvements were not costly.

Record reviews can also be useful for:

- Identifying health staff numbers and ratios and where they are working
- Registers can provide data on where patients live and their access to facilities
- Who is using health facilities when attendances are low, and any cultural factors involved
- Prescriptions can provide good data on use of drugs, injections, antibiotics, and generic drugs
- Case reviews can show whether treatment guidelines are being correctly followed

7.3 Making observations

This is a simple and quick method to document actual behaviour using an unstructured or structured checklist; for example, reviewing the condition of clinic rooms or obstetric facilities, observing how health workers relate to patients, or how well the laboratory or pharmacy are working. This is sometimes called 'management by walking around'.

A more structured approach can investigate if specific procedures are being performed according to standard treatment protocols and can also reveal the state of buildings, availability of drugs, presence of working and broken equipment, comfort of patient waiting areas, and privacy for patients. Observations can also help to understand why and how local communities and households appear to behave in certain ways, such as in disposing refuse, water hygiene, latrine use, cooking facilities, and hand washing. This can also be helpful when designing community health education messages.

For example, if procedures in health services and programmes are not being implemented correctly, do the guidelines need to be revised or is further in-service staff training necessary? Similar observations can be made with people living in local communities.

Structured observations

Structured observations involve starting by explaining the purpose to health workers and then to patients, and by asking for their permission to make these observations; remember, they are free to refuse. Their privacy and confidentiality must be respected. Introduce the purpose of the observation and reassure workers and patients, for example, that treatment guidelines are being reviewed for quality of care:

- Observe and listen to health workers and patients without interfering
- Use a written checklist and write down any observations in an unobtrusive manner
- Do not intervene if something is wrong unless it is serious or life-threatening
- Thank those observed and tell them they will not be personally quoted or identified in any reports

7.4 Patient facility exit interviews

It is important to know if people are satisfied with the quality of local services and how they feel they are being treated by the health staff. This can be assessed by interviewing patients as they leave clinics and asking them whether they are satisfied with how they were treated. They can also be asked to recall instructions on patient homecare and use of medicines. However, people using services are likely to say they are satisfied, and their answers can be biased, particularly if questions are asked by local health workers.

Conducting exit interviews

As patients are leaving a health facility, reassure patients about confidentiality and then question them using an agreed set of structured or unstructured questions, such as satisfaction with treatment, clinic waiting times, attitudes of health workers, understanding of health messages, use of prescribed medicines, and even any requests for unofficial payments or rewards. Bear the following in mind:

- To minimize bias the interviewer should not be a staff member or a locally well-known person
- Assess patients' ability to memorize and recall any instructions for prescribed medicines and on how to treat the condition at home. How clear were the health worker's instructions?
- Answers will be influenced by the patient's educational level, socio-economic status, exposure to similar previous health messages and health topics in the mass media

7.5 Key informant interviews

These interviews, also called in-depth interviews, are with people who are knowledgeable about local issues such as health managers, programme coordinators, community leaders, local administrators, financial personnel, and local opinion leaders. Teachers, religious leaders, and politicians are usually well-respected on local issues.

A variety of different key informant interviews are particularly useful for obtaining an in-depth understanding of community views, such as public perceptions about the quality of the health services, causes of dissatisfaction, and the best ways to provide the community with public information.

Performing interviews

Use an interview guide with a specific list of up to 12 questions. If possible, record interviews so they can be listened to again. Interviews are important to obtain answers to such questions as:

'What is your opinion on the costs to you of using local health services?'

- Explain the interview, conduct it in a private place, and give reassurances about confidentiality
- Most interviews take about one hour up to two hours. Voice-recording of interviews can be helpful if interviewees agree to this. If this is not possible, allow more time to write down the answers
- Listen carefully and avoid interruptions, although remember that some people may need help to focus on the issues
- Use an informal conversational approach and give reassurance on how the information will be used

Write down and/or record the answers accurately and obtain permission to do this before the interview. Finally, thank respondents for their time and reassure them about confidentiality.

7.6 Focus group discussions (FGD)

A focus group consists of a small sample of people brought together to discuss a topic or issue to ascertain the range and intensity of their views, beliefs, or explanations. These groups are often used to explore health-related perceptions of diseases and services and to test out questionnaires.

Focus groups are helpful in revealing people's health attitudes and their perceptions, knowledge, and behaviours, as well as their views on different health services. For instance, concerning the safe delivery of babies, one group of women might be those who have delivered in local health facilities, another who have not, and another group whose babies were delivered by their husbands. Other groups might be unmarried or newly married women, pregnant women wanting to deliver at home, or even a group of grandmothers.

FOCUS GROUPS CAN REVEAL PEOPLE'S BELIEFS AND ATTITUDES

FGDs involve the following:

- Start by forming small, selected groups of 6 to 12 people from the community who have an interest in the issue for discussion. A good focus group lasts about one to two hours.
- Group participants should be knowledgeable about the issues to be discussed and of similar age, gender, socio-economic status, and ethnicity. Different groups can discuss the same topic.
- A facilitator presents the issues and enables everyone to express themselves freely. They can also help avoid any one person dominating the group. An assistant can make notes and operate a recorder.

Begin by explaining the issue and then ask a general question such as 'Where do most women deliver their babies?' Followed by a more specific question like 'Why do you think most women deliver at home or in the health centre?' It is important that every group member is asked to contribute on the issue. It is best if the group talks together in a discussion rather than it being a question-and-answer session.

Questions help participants focus on the issue while the facilitator needs to gently steer the discussion in the required direction. Note-taking or recording is important in order to capture the main discussion points.

If necessary, probe for more detail, such as ask why do most mothers attend antenatal clinics but not as many deliver their babies in their local health facilities? What do they know about complications during delivery? What would encourage more pregnant mothers to be delivered by a trained midwife?

Make sure all the participants know when and where to meet. If necessary, provide refreshments. It is not usual to pay participants to attend.

Make notes on all the issues that aroused strong opinions and emotions, including anger and fear. Note what some people actually say so they can be quoted. Make a written record of the discussions. Finally, thank all participants and reassure them about confidentiality.

It is important to conduct more than one FGD if possible and it is best to stop when new groups appear to bring no more additional insights compared to those provided by earlier groups.

Table 7.2 shows what different groups of health workers believed were the main causes of the health problems experienced by local children. Poor levels of nutrition and poor parenting and education were identified, although no group of workers believed their health care had been inadequate.

Table 7.2 Use of ten focus groups of health workers to explore their perceptions on the main causes of children's health problems

Group	Poor nutrition	Poor Parenting	Poor Education	Poverty	Diseases	Inadequate Health care
1	XXX	XX			X	
2		XXX		XX	XX	X
3	XX	XXX	X			
4	XX		XXX	X	X	X
5	X	XXX	XX		X	
6	XXX		XX	X	XX	
7	XXX	XX	XX	X		
8	XXX	X		XX		
9	XXX	XX		X		
10	XX	XXX			X	

Ranking of problem: high = XXX; medium = XX; low = X

7.7 Participatory rural appraisal

This rapid method involves investigators and community members working together to explain issues primarily from the community's perspective. It was developed by social and agricultural specialists working in rural areas. People describe, map, and illustrate their lives with images, objects, and symbols to produce a visual representation of their community. For instance, members might draw a map showing health facilities, households, and local health problems. This approach can reveal how seasonal changes can affect health services and programmes and how disease patterns can change throughout the year. A month-by-month calendar can show any seasonal changes in more detail.

Maps and calendars can help facilitators discuss community priorities and what help and changes the community members would like to see. Repeating this exercise in different parts of the district will provide a wider picture about priorities and planners can use the findings in their local health planning.

7.8 Triangulation and analysing data

Qualitative investigations aim to give insights into the main reasons for particular beliefs and behaviours by making observations that cannot easily be expressed in numbers or by percentages. Analysis looks for common perceptions, beliefs, and themes. For instance, the health problems for children can be summarized using key words such as malnutrition, poor parenting, inadequate education, poverty, diseases, and inadequate health care. The strength of people's answers can be indicated in a summary chart (see Table 7.3) and findings from different methods can suggest what further actions are required.

Analysis is best done by hand, although computer programmes are available for the analysis of large qualitative surveys. It is important to analyse how often the same issue recurs in different discussions, interviews, and focus groups. In written reports it is good practice to use anonymous quotes to express common views but avoid being too selective or using sensational statements. And do not identify individual participants.

Triangulation is when the same findings and conclusions are found by using different qualitative approaches. For instance, direct observation might reveal that patients are not being treated with respect by health staff and that this is linked to their apparent lack of confidence in their work. Key informants might confirm that health workers are often rude to patients, and this might also be reported by different focus groups. These findings by different methods and different groups can be triangulated together and provide stronger evidence that the findings are indeed correct.

GOOD TRIANGULATION PROVIDES STRONGER EVIDENCE

8

Health Surveys

8.1 Using surveys

Surveys use **descriptive epidemiology** to ask what are the health risks, diseases, or events and their frequency, and who is involved, where, and when? What is the rate of utilization of particular interventions? What is the distribution and use of different services?

Surveys may be necessary to collect local data on the delivery, access, quality, and coverage of particular health interventions by the services and programmes, or by being involved in a national health and demographic survey. These surveys are also carried out to collect data on risk behaviours such as smoking or unsafe sexual practices or to establish the frequency of chronic diseases such as hypertension, diabetes, or blindness. Surveys can also be used to assess the effectiveness of particular health intervention programmes and help establish base-line data for new initiatives.

Surveys are useful for:

- Estimating incidence or prevalence of important diseases, such as malaria and malnutrition, and risk factors such as obesity, diabetes, and raised blood pressure
- Screening population groups for treatment of important diseases, care of pregnant mothers, young children, schoolchildren, or plantation and factory workers

- Collecting health information about households and their members, such as for excreta disposal, seasonal nutritional security, food preferences, and health-seeking behaviours
- Finding out about local beliefs and customs, such as for breastfeeding and family planning
- Understanding the uptake of new interventions, such as for Covid-19, including hand washing, physical distancing, wearing of face masks, and uptake of vaccines
- Evaluating the effectiveness of the health services, such as for antenatal attendance, immunization coverage, and utilization of outpatient clinics

When planning a survey local staff may need expert advice. Alternatively, they may be involved in the preparation of a protocol for national studies when their cooperation and involvement can be essential. For example, Figure 8.1 shows how health staff might be involved in a national nutrition survey and what might be expected from them.

Local staff may also need to organize their own epidemiological surveys, for example to estimate coverage of immunization or antenatal services, or to find out why some households are not cooperating with the antimalarial spray team, or to screen schoolchildren for helminthic infections. It is good ethical practice to encourage public trust and cooperation by offering a health service to all participants who are taking part in a survey.

NO SURVEY WITHOUT A SOME SERVICES

Surveys involve the following main stages. The first is to clarify the need for the survey and then to state the objectives. Next come questions about sampling and details of which methods to use, followed by the organization and

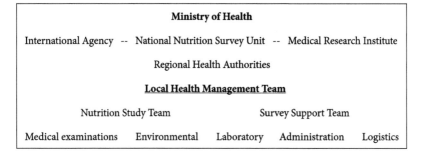

Figure 8.1 Possible local involvement in a national nutrition survey

implementation of the survey itself. Analysis of the data and interpretation of the findings then lead to conclusions and recommendations. And finally, how will the information be used to improve local health planning and disease control programmes?

Main steps in an epidemiological survey are:

1. Identify and clarify the problem for investigation
2. Review published and unpublished literature
3. Seek advice and consult experts
4. Determine the priority of the problem
5. Formulate the hypothesis
6. Determine research questions, objectives, sample, and methods
7. Train interviewers and organize the survey
8. Collect and analyse the data
9. Interpret the findings
10. Write the report with conclusions and recommendations
11. Disseminate and communicate the findings
12. Incorporate the findings into local planning

8.2 Cross-sectional and longitudinal surveys

Cross-sectional surveys examine people at one point in time and therefore mainly provide prevalence data. They are useful for infectious diseases and conditions that last a relatively long time such as malnutrition, leprosy, human immunodeficiency virus/acquired immunodeficiency syndrome (HIV/AIDS), health-risk behaviours, and serological surveys for evidence of immunity due to previous infections. The 'point in time' can be several weeks or months, providing that the frequency of the conditions under investigation do not change during this period. Cross-sectional surveys are less useful for short-duration and rare diseases or events. Prevalence data can be more difficult to interpret than incidence data.

For a disease or event that shows considerable seasonal fluctuation, a careful choice has to be made about the most appropriate time of year to undertake the survey, and how quickly to collect the data.

> **CROSS-SECTIONAL SURVEYS COLLECT MAINLY PREVALENCE DATA**

Longitudinal surveys collect information about all new cases or events occurring over a period of time and therefore collect incidence data, such as new cases of measles or tuberculosis (TB) or number of pregnant mothers attending the antenatal clinic for the first time. The time period for collecting the incidence data must be defined. Longitudinal surveys may be organized in a similar way to surveillance for new cases of communicable diseases.

Health staff should be able to organize their own cross-sectional surveys for common problems, but longitudinal surveys are more complicated and are mainly used in health and research studies. Some incidence data can be collected by repeated cross-sectional surveys and asking people about events in the two or more weeks prior to the survey. Repeated cross-sectional surveys in the same population can also be used to estimate the incidence of a disease or event. However, this is possible only for chronic diseases that cannot come and then go undetected between the two surveys. Cross-sectional surveys for chronic diseases are rarely repeated again in less than one year. A repeat survey is usually best carried out in the same month as the initial survey to help avoid the effects of seasonal differences and any changes that might affect the frequency of the disease or event.
Cross-sectional surveys are useful for:

- Collecting information on prevalence
- Descriptive information, screening, and estimating use of services
- Common conditions of long average duration
- Quick and easily organized surveys
- Estimating incidence if two cross-sectional surveys are carried out

8.3 Survey objectives

It is important to be clear and precise about what questions are being asked and only then to decide if a cross-sectional survey will provide the answers. Objectives help determine the required population sample and identify the appropriate survey methods. Common faults in surveys are a lack of clarity in the precise question and poor formulation of the objectives.

Question: What is the prevalence of malnutrition among villagers in this district and are there any gender differences?

Table 8.1 Distribution of hookworm-infected subjects by haemoglobin level

Haemoglobin level	Hookworm infection		Total % with hookworm
	Present Absent		
Less than 9.0 g/100 ml			
9.0 g/100 ml or more			
Total % with anaemia			

Objective: Determine the prevalence of mild, moderate, and severe malnutrition among male and female children aged 12–36 months living in the district.

At an early stage it is useful to set out **dummy tables**. For example, to study haemoglobin level and the presence of hookworm infection by age and gender is shown in sample Tables 8.1 and 8.2. These help to clarify what survey data need to be collected.

8.4 Selecting the sample

All the people in the district or local area of concern are the **reference population**, but it is unusual to investigate every individual. It is more common to select a sample, called the **sample population**. To help avoid selection bias due to poor sampling, each person in the reference population should have an equal

Table 8.2 Distribution of haemoglobin levels for villagers by age and sex

Haemoglobin level (g/100 ml)	Age group (years)										Total
	0–4		5–14		15–44		45–64		65+		
	M	F	M	F	M	F	M	F	M	F	
< 6.0											
7.0											
8.0											
9.0											
10.0											
11.0											
12.0											
13.0 =>											
Total											

chance of being included in the survey. The sample population will then probably be representative of the larger reference population. Unrepresentative and incorrect sampling are common faults with surveys.

> **All INDIVIDUALS SHOULD HAVE AN EQUAL CHANCE OF BEING IN THE SAMPLE**

Studying the whole population would need much more effort and money and large studies can also introduce their own errors and biases. Sometimes studying the entire population is unavoidable, for instance when information is needed on all possible cases during an epidemic or when selecting a group of people would be seen as discriminating against others.

It is important to define which people are to be surveyed, for example which sex, age group, occupation, and area. Samples keep the survey work down to a minimum while also obtaining meaningful and representative data.

There are two main methods of drawing a sample, random and systematic. For statistical reasons, **random sampling** is more likely to provide a representative sample but a **systematic sample** may be more convenient and easier to adopt in practice.

Drawing a simple random sample:

- What is the **sample unit**? This can be a person, household, or village, as appropriate
- List all sampling units from which the sample will be drawn. This is the sampling frame
- Decide on the number of units to be chosen randomly from this frame. This is the **sample size** and is divided by the total number of available units in the sampling frame to give the sampling fraction
- Choose the required number of units from the sampling frame by a random method to ensure that each unit has an equal chance of being selected and included in the survey. This can be done either by using a table of random numbers or by drawing lots (see Annex Two)

Choosing a systematic sample:

- Start by choosing the first unit randomly
- Select the next units in a systematic manner, such as every fifth person on a list, every third hospital admission, or every tenth house on adjacent streets
- Different random starting units may be selected to give several clusters

A **cluster sample** may be used in a stratified sample when random sampling would be costly and time-consuming. This relies on randomly selecting clusters of villages or households and then including all people in the survey or taking a further random sample of people from the villages of households or individuals.

A cluster sample can be used to collect information on a common variable or condition. Using a cluster of 30 people within 7 households is an established technique that was originally developed for estimating immunization coverage amongst young children. It is now often used for descriptive cross-sectional surveys focusing on relatively common conditions or variables. It is important that the variable or condition is common as this method is not accurate for rare conditions and is unsuitable for measuring mortality and some health status indicators due to the small numbers involved. Cluster samples have several advantages including being convenient, having a simple sample frame, people are grouped together, community acceptance may be high, local leaders can be involved, and feedback can be simpler.

> **CLUSTER SAMPLES ARE OFTEN USED FOR CONVENIENCE AND LOW COSTS**

8.5 Calculating sample size

To determine the required sample size some previous estimates of prevalence are necessary. Cross-sectional surveys work best when the presumed prevalence is believed to be in the mid-range for the condition or event being investigated. Provided the sample is truly random, the larger the sample the more reliable the estimated prevalence rate will be, although using a larger but biased sample will probably not improve the accuracy of data.

The size of sample needed for a prevalence survey depends upon the accuracy required and the actual presumed prevalence of the condition itself. For example, leprosy and TB may have a prevalence of about 1 per 100 or 10 per 1,000 people. In a sample of 100 people, therefore, only 1 case would be expected and there is a reasonable chance that no cases at all would be observed. Such a small sample is unlikely to give an accurate estimate of the prevalence of leprosy or TB. Even in a sample of 1,000 people only 10 cases might be expected. For a more common condition such as urinary schistosomiasis with a known prevalence of, say, 30%, a sample of 100–200 people would give a reasonably accurate prevalence rate. A sample of 1,000 is not necessary.

If the sample is correctly selected, the larger it is the closer the survey estimate of prevalence is likely to be to the true prevalence in the whole community. However, smaller samples require less time, cost less, quality control and supervision will be easier, and small samples can ensure a better accuracy and repeatability of the data collected.

The required sample size is the smallest one that will give an acceptable level of accuracy. Table 8.3 shows the minimum sample sizes for various levels of expected prevalence and specified margins of sampling error for the estimated prevalence. It may be possible to quantify the error associated with the particular sampling method.

Table 8.3 provides a guide to the sample sizes required for various presumed prevalence rates. If the expected rate of a particular condition or event is about 40% in the overall population, the rate in a random sample of 50 people can vary widely between 26% and 55%. If the sample size is increased to 200, this range is reduced but only to 33% and 47%. There is greater accuracy in enlarging the sample of 50 to 200 but there is not much more accuracy with a larger sample of, say, 500 subjects which would involve a lot more work.

A sample of 100–200 subjects for a common condition will often be sufficient for most planning and management purposes. If greater accuracy is required for a low prevalence condition or a rare event then a much larger sample size will be needed. For a more detailed discussion on estimating sample size, see Annex Three.

8.6 Response rate

Even with well-chosen samples, surveys can still give misleading results if a high proportion of the selected sample of individuals or households is not seen or contacted or refuses to answer questions. This is called the **non-response rate**. Bias can be introduced by including those who are seen in the analysis while leaving out the non-responders who are not included. For instance, a survey in a rural area carried out during the day might miss men and women working in agriculture or in factories. Problems of poor sampling and poor response rates apply equally to all surveys.

To reduce the non-response rate it is necessary to see at least 80% of the original sample and to follow up all non-responders at least once.

FOLLOW UP ALL NON-RESPONDERS AT LEAST ONCE

Table 8.3 Survey sample size according to expected prevalence rates

Previous estimates of prevalence (%)	Size of sample				
	50	100	200	500	1000
	Probable range for estimates of prevalence rate %				
1	—	0–5	0.1–4	0.3– 3	0.5–2
5	—	2–11	2–9	3– 8	4–7
10	03–22	05–18	6–15	7–13	8–12
20	10–34	13–29	15–26	16–24	18–23
30	18–45	21–40	24–37	26–35	27–33
40	26–55	30–50	33–47	35–45	37–43
50	36–64	40–60	43–57	45–55	47–53
60	45–74	50–70	53–67	55–65	57–63
70	55–82	60–79	63–76	65–74	67–73
80	66–90	71–87	74–85	76–84	77–82
90	78–97	82–95	85–94	87–93	88–92

Non-response in surveys of common conditions can be critical when subjects who are seen may be different from those who are not seen. For instance, when the survey is investigating a sensitive disease or event such as HIV infection, alcohol consumption, or family planning, subjects may be elusive, give evasive answers, or even decide not to attend. This can lead to false estimates of prevalence. Conversely people may respond if they believe they may gain by attending, as in malnutrition surveys linked to distribution of free food supplements or financial incentives.

8.7 Accuracy of measurements

It is also very important to consider other non-sampling errors. For instance, measurements can easily be inaccurate and this is most often due to the survey staff and not because of unreliable subjects or faulty instruments. This is known as **observer error**, a non-sampling error. Instrument errors can be avoided by checking instruments regularly, such as adjusting the zero reading on weighing scales.

> OBSERVERS AND INTERVIEWERS ARE THE MAIN SOURCE OF
> NON-SAMPLING ERRORS AND INACCURACIES

Other common observer errors are due to the way interviewers ask questions and the faulty recording of information on portable devices, record forms, or questionnaires. Measurements can easily be inaccurate, and this is often due to the survey staff and not due to there being unreliable subjects or faulty instruments.

Inaccuracies and errors can be reduced by carefully training all staff and by re-interviewing and spot-checking that the methods are being correctly used, such as following all agreed guidelines for weighing infants or how to ask questions in a questionnaire:

- Use 'blind' methods if possible where neither the subject nor observer are aware of why the data are being collected. If they know this it can lead them to bias their answers or their techniques
- Ask staff to sign their name against a case history, physical examination, measurement, or laboratory test to make it clear who performed them and ensure accountability
- Review all questionnaires and records at the end of each day for inaccuracies and inconsistencies
- Check all instruments daily, such as weighing scales being checked with a 10 kg weight

Ensure careful supervision at all times to detect any possible and systematic errors early, and provide daily feedback to staff and discuss any problems as a team.

8.8 Questionnaires

Questionnaires may look simple but in fact a good questionnaire can be difficult to design. They are used to collect information, usually with an interviewer-administered questionnaire on a **hand-held portable device** or on paper, asking about what activities people have been doing, their social and economic status, what foods they eat, any recent illnesses, births and deaths, and where they go to attend health services. Each question needs to be simple, clear, and non-threatening.

This information is often difficult or impossible to obtain in any other way. For example, it is easier to ask people where they get their domestic water supply than to observe them fetching their water. However, remember that such information is what people say they do and this may be very different from what they actually do!

Some common problems with questionnaires are:

- Poorly designed questions, which are unclear, badly worded, or actually ask more than one question
- Leading questions can influence responses and may suggest correct or incorrect answers
- Too many questions can be tiresome or boring for both interviewers and subjects
- Quality of data collected is often inversely proportional to the length of the questionnaire
- Sensitive and personal questions may produce evasive answers; first ask general questions and later the more sensitive ones
- Subjects may not remember events that occurred previously and a recall period of two weeks is often the maximum that can be relied upon, except for major events such as births, deaths, or hospital admissions

It is extremely important to pilot test questionnaires for any mistakes and difficulties before using them in any investigations (see Figure 8.2).

Interviewers should record what the subjects say or use pre-coded answers but should not re-interpret the subject's answers. And allow 15–20 minutes for an interview, including basic questions for name, age, and sex, so that 3–4 people can be interviewed per hour.

Avoid non-standardized questions, often stated in one language but translated and delivered in another local language. Test all translated questionnaires by translating them with one set of people and then back-translating by another group. This highlights misunderstandings, problems, and discrepancies.

Interviewees may wonder why the questions are being asked and who else will be given the data or information. This can lead to suspicion and biased answers. Before starting the questionnaire, the interviewers should provide a reasonable and full explanation about the survey, with strong assurances on confidentiality and the subsequent use of the information.

PILOT-TEST ALL QUESTIONNAIRES AND RECORD FORMS

After designing a questionnaire, it is essential to **pilot test** it using interviewers and a small group of people who are similar to those for whom it is intended. This is to correct any mistakes or ambiguities and to train all interviewers in the agreed final version. Role-playing by the interviewers under the critical eye of colleagues is useful way to ensure a standardized technique by all the interviewers.

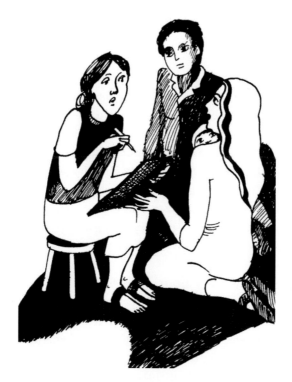

Figure 8.2 Interviewer pilot testing a questionnaire before use in a household survey

Reproduced with permission from Vaughan, J Patrick, Morrow, Richard H, and World Health Organization, Manual of epidemiology for district health management, World Health Organization; Geneva, Switzerland, Copyright © 1989

It is also important to demonstrate the **validity** of all questionnaires. For example, in a survey of two villages in an area endemic for schistosomiasis people were asked: 'Do you have blood in your urine?' Urine samples were also examined for eggs of *S. haematobium*, a helminthic infestation of the bladder and urinary tract. In one village the question was considered offensive by the women, leading to marked under-reporting by them compared to the findings in the urine samples. In another village there was no such taboo and there was good agreement between the interview and urine results for both men and women. Without the laboratory test the questionnaire results might have led to the conclusion that in the first village, schistosomiasis was more common in men than women.

Interviewers can also influence how subjects answer questions, which should be asked in a neutral and non-threatening manner and without indicating the answers. Interviewers should not express agreement or disagreement nor pleasure or distaste with any answers. Neutrality only comes with careful training.

Health workers often make poor interviewers as they can have difficulties in remaining neutral and find it hard to reframe from giving their own interpretation or advice. Interviewers are often recruited, therefore, from non-health staff such as teachers, extension workers, or secondary-school children. In many cultures, especially when asking about sensitive subjects like family planning and childbirth, it is best for women to interview women and men to interview men. The interviewer's gender can influence responses.

THOROUGHLY TRAIN AND SUPERVISE ALL INTERVIEWERS

8.9 Choosing variables

Variables are characteristics that are measured either numerically (e.g. age) or in categories (e.g. absence or presence of diabetes or hypertension), and each one must be reproducible for them to be useful. In surveys it is important to use standardized methods for all variables. Questionnaires should only include relevant variables that are needed in the subsequent analysis; all other non-essential questions can be discarded. Each item needs to be justified, so include as many variables as needed at the start but finally have as few as possible.

When deciding on which variables to include it is best to first start with a comprehensive list and then review each variable in detail to see whether the collected data for that particular variable will be used in the ultimate analysis. Dummy tables (see Table 8.3) can be helpful in identifying the essential variables.

DISCARD ANY UNNECESSARY OR IRRELEVANT VARIABLES

When the variables have been chosen, next plan how to measure them under survey conditions. Each variable should have a good definition and a reliable method to measure them objectively.

All variables and cases must be clearly defined since illnesses and health behaviours often have different meanings for different people. For example, a common cold may be interpreted as influenza. These differences can lead to data that are not repeatable and probably not valid. Malaria needs to be defined, such as a child with fever and chills, or one with an enlarged spleen or the presence of *Plasmodium* parasites in a blood film, or a combination of all these different criteria.

Variables should have standardized and simple operational definitions so that they can easily be applied. Using detailed techniques, such as those in clinical medicine, is often not practical in surveys.

8.10 Including socio-demographic variables

Many variables can be associated with health status and to understand health inequalities it is important to analyse data by age, gender, ethnicity, and marital status, as well as by education, occupation, and household wealth. For instance, place of residence can be recorded in different ways, such as urban or rural, and for larger cities as residential, slum, and shanty town, and for rural areas by district, subdistrict, village, or local settlement. Smartphones or tablets can be used to collect data and record household GPS coordinates to analyse health indicators using small area statistics.

Education of the head of household, or for child health surveys the child's mother, is usually recorded as years of schooling completed with a pass grade. Alternatively educational level may be recorded as none, incomplete primary, primary, incomplete secondary, secondary, or tertiary. Categories will depend on the schooling in each country and the distribution of the population. It is best to have at least three different groups with each one having a sufficient sample size. For example, if the number of people with complete secondary education is too small then incomplete secondary, secondary, and tertiary may be combined into one group.

Occupation can be hard to measure accurately, given that people may have several different occupations at the same time and change their work during different seasons or have had different employments in the past compared today. In some societies, the majority of people have the same general occupation, such as agriculture, fishing, or street vendor. Such broad occupational groupings are often not used as a stratification variable in routine surveys.

Household wealth can be assessed by using an asset index based on household goods (e.g. radio, television, smartphones, etc.) and on building characteristics (e.g. materials used in the floor, walls, and roof, and presence of piped water and electricity, etc.). Many countries have such indices included in regular maternal and child health surveys, such as demographic and health surveys (DHS) or multiple indicator cluster surveys (MICS). Using a statistical method called principal component analysis, a single index measure can be derived that ranks all sample households into five wealth quintiles groups, from the poorest 20% to the wealthiest 20%. District teams can request help with this approach from epidemiology or statistics departments in a national university or research organization.

Results shown by wealth quintile can be particularly important and often show considerable variation between poor and wealthier people. Data from health surveys on indicators of inequalities should be disaggregated and reported in tables, figures, and graphs. The minimum set of stratification variables should include age, sex, place of residence, ethnicity (if relevant in the district), and at least one socio-economic indicator such as education, occupation, or wealth quintiles.

8.11 Repeatability and validity

It is important that findings are **repeatable** even though simplified techniques may miss a small percentage of cases, or even include a few non-cases. Repeatability examines whether the methods when repeated again obtain the same results. **Validity** refers to the extent to which the test is capable of correctly diagnosing the presence or absence of a condition or disease or event. Repeatability and validity are mainly determined by which methods are used (see Annex Four).

Repeatability of the data is determined when measurements are repeated in the same population using the same methods. Even simple measurements may have substantial errors caused by observer error, non-observer and experimental errors, instrument error, and those related to test performance.

The more reliable the method, the more repeatable the data are likely to be. If variability leads to random fluctuations in values above and below the true mean, a relationship that actually exists may be missed although making false conclusions are unlikely. If there is bias with a consistent over- or underestimate from the true value (a bias) the readings will be consistently be lower or higher than they actually should be. This can lead to faulty conclusions. **Repeatability of a measurement can be affected by:**

- Observer variation occurs when a single person (intra-observer variation) or different people (inter-observer variation) carry out the measurements; for example, when the same or different technician examines blood slides for malaria parasites or when different doctors measure blood pressure

- Subject variation is where responses to a question may vary and be affected by the subject's own motivations and beliefs or be influenced by how and where the interviews take place
- Instrument and method variation is when some instruments and methods are more unreliable than others

8.12 Validity of screening tests

Validity refers to the extent to which the test correctly diagnoses the presence or absence of a condition or disease or event. High validity requires good definitions. Epidemiology often uses preselected diagnostic criteria to answer the question: 'Does this individual in the population sample have the condition I am studying or not?'

Testing for the validity and repeatability of different methods is crucial. Diagnostic criteria may require standardized interviews and physical and laboratory examinations, as well as more elaborate examinations such as electrocardiography for heart disease or histopathology for skin cancers.

The **validity** of screening tests is usually judged on their **sensitivity, specificity, and predictive value**. A test has a sensitivity of 90% if it correctly gives a positive result in 90% of people who actually do have the disease or condition. This means that 10% of patients who do have the disease will not have a positive test. These are **false negatives** (see Annex Four).

A test has a specificity of 90% if it correctly gives a negative result in 90% of people who do not have the disease. There will be 10% who, although negative, are actually designated as **false positives**.

The positive **predictive value** of a test measures the likelihood that a person who has tested positive actually has the disease. It is an important measure in determining a test's usefulness under actual service or survey conditions. This greatly depends on the prevalence of the disease or condition and on the sensitivity and specificity of the test. The lower the prevalence rate the lower the positive predictive value which will result in more false positive results.

The user of a test may also need to make a choice between different tests based on their **predictive value**. This is the most important measure for determining the test's usefulness under 'field' conditions. It depends on the prevalence of the disease or condition as well as the test's sensitivity and specificity.

Different prevalence rates affect the positive predictive value. For example, for a diagnostic test with a sensitivity of 95% used with a condition that has a prevalence of 20%, the positive predictive value for a positive result is 83%.

However, if the same test is used in a population where the disease or event prevalence is only 1%, the positive predictive value falls to only 16%. This means that of all positives found by the screening test only 16%, or about one in six, are true positives. This shows that even with a test with high sensitivity and specificity the positive predictive value can fall from 83% to 16% when the prevalence drops from 20% to 1%. This same situation can occur when a disease control or eradication programme has been successfully implemented and the prevalence falls to a lower level. For instance, this can occur in successful malaria and onchocerciasis control programmes.

Repeatability, validity, and predictive value are considered in more detail in Annex Four.

8.13 Ethical issues for surveys

Ethical issues are important even before deciding to undertake a survey. Major ethical issues concern large scale research studies while surveys undertaken as a part of the work of local health services are usually viewed less rigorously. Chapter 16 and Annex Five have more details on the ethical issues.

In countries with less well-developed health services the surveyed population often expects some help with their health problems if they cooperate. Offering a health service should be a part of any survey. For instance, people suffering from a disease or who have missed out on a preventive health measure, such as immunization, should be referred to an appropriate local clinic or health facility.

In population-based research, it is often not clear who can or should give consent for the study or investigation, such as participants, family members, or husbands in some countries, or community chiefs or district manager:

- Study participants should give informed consent based on their own understanding of the full information provided by the researchers
- At community level, local authorities (e.g. chiefs, village or cell leaders, council chairpersons) must be informed about the research and give their approval for the study to go ahead. However, participation is ultimately decided by individuals under the principles of autonomy and informed consent. Leaders can support research taking place in their jurisdiction but they cannot give consent on behalf of other people (Figure 8.3)

Informed consent is an important issue. It requires that individuals are given the full reasons for the survey and any investigations. Each individual

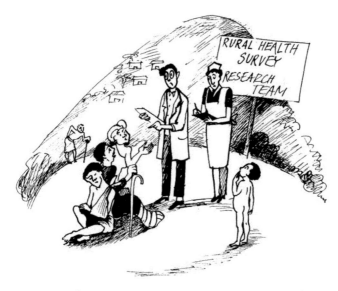

"I'M SORRY, WE CAME ONLY TO COUNT YOU....."

Figure 8.3 No survey without a health care service

Reproduced with permission from Vaughan, J Patrick, Morrow, Richard H, and World Health Organization, Manual of epidemiology for district health management, World Health Organization; Geneva, Switzerland, Copyright © 1989

in the survey must be fully informed about the reason for the survey so they can give their consent or not. They should also know that they are free to decline to participate. More care is needed when a potentially harmful procedure is used, such as providing a non-standard drug with unpleasant or dangerous side effects or an invasive procedure is used such as collecting blood samples or throat swabs. For well established procedures it may be sufficient to brief community leaders and follow this with an announcement that allows people to withdraw. See Box 16.2 for guidelines for informed consent.

Participants may be asked to sign and declare their agreement to participate in the survey. However, in many cultures, people might be very reluctant to give any written consent. Keeping data confidential and anonymous is also very important. Information is given in confidence and must not be passed to third parties. In addition, no individuals should be identified in the analysis or in subsequent reports. Individual information contained in the records should never be passed on to other people or organizations without the subject's consent.

> ## INFORMED CONSENT AND CONFIDENTIALITY ARE
> ## VERY IMPORTANT

Serious ethical issues may also arise when survey investigators do not feed back their findings and recommendations to the survey participants themselves or do not publicize or publish their findings and recommendations for use by health planners. They may rightly be asked, 'So, why was the survey done at all?'

Such difficult ethical issues should be discussed with community leaders, senior health staff, and with research institutes for their comments, advice, and permission. See Annex Five for more details on population-based research studies.

8.14 Survey methods checklist

In order to avoid problems in carrying out surveys or in interpreting the findings, particular attention must be given to:

- Using only clear and quantified objectives
- Good definitions of cases and events
- Proper sampling procedures and adequate sample size
- Investigating low response and high refusal rates
- Avoiding bias by using standardized techniques and good equipment
- Using well-designed, tested, and translated questionnaires
- Supervising and training all interviewers
- Conducting good pilot trials of methods, questionnaires, and equipment
- Practising consistent use of methods throughout the survey
- Using good communications with the population on permission, consent, and confidentiality
- Follow ethical guidelines (see Annex Five for more details)

9

Health Quantitative Studies

9.1 Observational studies

Although district health staff are unlikely to undertake health quantitative studies (other than cross-sectional surveys) themselves, it is important that they understand the concepts and principles involved as these are widely used in epidemiology. In addition, district health workers may well be invited to collaborate with academic colleagues in large epidemiological studies and to provide data for national studies.

Cross-sectional health surveys aim to measure disease frequency while this chapter focuses on designs to test hypotheses using observational studies that make use of **analytical epidemiology**. These attempt to analyse the causes or determinants of health problems and diseases or events by testing hypotheses about what caused the problem, why it is continuing, what are its consequences, as well as how it might be controlled. This approach looks for statistical associations between exposures to possible causes and any subsequent health outcomes.

Two types of observational studies, **case-control** and **cohort** study designs, are commonly used in epidemiological studies and in clinical investigations. However, to obtain valid findings they need to be carefully designed and implemented carefully in order to avoid various sources of bias and errors, including in the sample selection of participants and biases due to observers and measurements.

Case-control studies are an analytical epidemiological study that compare cases of a particular condition with suitable control subjects, looking at the frequency of associated factors (often called 'risk factors') in the two groups. These studies are used to test hypotheses about aetiology, such as the links between lung cancer and cigarette smoking. These retrospective studies look backwards in the life of the cases for possible earlier exposures in order to test a hypothesis about possible associations, although they cannot themselves be used to identify a causal association.

Cohort studies examine a well-defined group of people who have had a common experience or exposure and are then followed up for the incidence of new diseases or events. A birth cohort is people born during a particular period of time, often one year. These studies use a prospective design to observe both exposed and non-exposed groups over a future period of time and record the incidence of the outcome or disease of interest in each group. No active interventions are implemented in either group. Cohort studies are useful for identifying possible causal associations because they observe both the exposed and the not-exposed over time to identify future outcomes.

9.2 Case-control studies

These are retrospective studies because they look backwards from the disease or outcome to a possible earlier exposure to a potential cause. They provide a relatively quick epidemiological method to investigate associations between a previous exposure and a possible disease outcome, such as a history of hepatitis infection and a disease outcome such as liver cirrhosis, or for behavioural risk factors like smoking and subsequent lung cancer. They compare the frequency of past exposure in the cases with that in controls to compare both frequencies. The odds ratio or risk can then be calculated.

These studies start by carefully selecting the cases according to clear criteria, including that they should be as representative as possible of all the cases in the general population. It is often preferable to select only new cases although previous cases, for instance those recorded in a cancer registry, can be included. New cases diagnosed in hospitals or clinics is often used as a starting point. For long-standing conditions such as congenital abnormalities it is more acceptable to include cases from a specialized register. The exposure status of the cases and controls are retrospectively determined after their inclusion in the study. For instance, this may be with a questionnaire for exposure to particular foods, previous employments, or by using biochemical markers such as lead or antibody levels in blood samples.

In typical case-control studies (also known as case/non-case studies), controls are selected from people who do not have the outcome but who must also be as representative as possible of the population from which the cases were selected. Cases can be matched with control subjects for some variables, such as age and sex, and if possible by other factors such as location and employment, but it is impractical to match for more than four variables. Over-matching is best avoided because any variables used for matching, or variables related to these, cannot be studied as risk factors as by definition their frequency will be similar in cases and controls. Control subjects and matches should also be as representative as possible of the general population from which the cases came. To avoid bias it is best that controls are selected from a similar group of people and not selected from an easily identifiable or convenient healthy population sub-group, such as healthy workers or students.

Case-control design is shown in Box 9.1. The choice of the number of cases and controls depends on the estimated incidence of the outcome in the general population. A rare outcome with a low incidence may require a large number of cases and two or more controls for every case that is included.

The association between an exposure and the outcome—called the odds ratio and sometimes the relative risk—can be measured approximately using the odds ratio, which is the ratio among cases compared to the controls. The attributable risk is unreliable when the actual incidence is unknown for the disease or event, and neither can it be accurately determined.

The value for the OR can be tested for significance (p value) using the chi square test, and 95% confidence intervals must always be presented.

Box 9.1 Design for a case-control study

		Cases	Population
	⟸ Time		
Exposed		a	
Not Exposed		c	
		Controls	Population
Exposed		b	
Not exposed		d	

Table 9.1 Odds ratio between the exposure and outcome

		Exposure		
		Yes	No	Total
Disease or outcome	Yes	a	b	a + b
	No	c	d	c + d
	Total	a + c	b + d	a + b + c + d
Odds ratio (OR) is:	$= \dfrac{a \times d}{b \times c}$			

A case-control design can be used in an epidemic to help determine a source of exposure, see Section 7.6.

9.3 Cohort studies

These are follow-up studies based on longitudinal observations on two or more groups which allow for the measurement of disease incidence. Cohort studies are useful for identifying possible causal associations and in typical prospective cohorts the outcome is detected after the possible exposure (see Box 9.2).

Cohort studies begin with people who are free of the disease or outcome of interest and who are then classified into at least two groups: those exposed to a potential cause and those not exposed. Both the exposed and not-exposed groups are then observed prospectively, maybe over a long period of time, in order to record the incidence of the outcome or disease in each group. No active health interventions are used in either group.

The basic design is shown in Box 9.2. This methodology was used in the classical studies investigating exposure to cigarette smoking and its association with lung cancer. Cohort studies can provide the best information on both the relative individual risk for developing the disease or event and for the attributable risks for different levels of exposures. Other studies using this approach have included cohort studies for antenatal and child health care, risk factors for cardiovascular and cerebrovascular diseases, and occupational exposures to work hazards such as coal mining and asbestos.

These studies usually require long periods of observation in order to detect a sufficient number of new incident cases and to collect the best data. This can make these studies both prolonged and expensive on staff time and resources. The cohort design is best used when the incidence of interest is reasonably

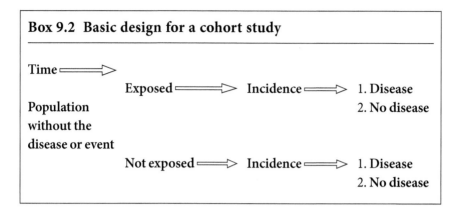

Box 9.2 Basic design for a cohort study

Time ⟹

Population without the disease or event

Exposed ⟹ Incidence ⟹ 1. Disease
2. No disease

Not exposed ⟹ Incidence ⟹ 1. Disease
2. No disease

common because studies on rare diseases or events require large samples and long periods of time for observation. If acute exposures are followed soon afterwards by the outcome of interest, a causal relationship may be obvious, and therefore intense and prolonged study is unnecessary.

Cohort studies usually measure incidence using person-time incidence in the population at risk over the observation time period which is divided by the number of person-time units, such as years observed to give the incidence rate as episodes for 1,000 persons over a time period of years or a lifetime. This measure is often also used in cancer studies.

The above description refers to prospective cohort studies. Retrospective cohort studies are also possible which rely on existing records to classify exposure in the past, prior to occurrence of the disease outcome. For example, a study of all children born in a district can be classified according to their birth weight using hospital records from a previous year and children who died are then identified using death registration systems. The risk of infant mortality may then be estimated for different birth weight categories.

Cohort studies can also be a good design for examining routine data sources such as death certificates, disease registries, and hospital case histories, as well as for additional data on morbidity and mortality for a range of possible previous exposures. Population-based cohort studies have the added advantage that data can be examined for many different possible exposures and risk factors.

The value of existing cohort longitudinal data can also be expanded when other previous exposures can be included in a **nested case-control study**. Typically, this involves comparing characteristics of cases diagnosed during the follow-up period with a sample of non-cases, rather than with the full original cohort. These studies are particularly useful when obtaining data on possible exposures is expensive, for example when using genetic or biochemical tests. Because there are usually many more non-cases than cases, nested studies avoid testing a large number of non-cases, which statistically would be inefficient. The collected data can be used to test further ideas about possible associations and to investigate for possible causation. The risk ratio, odds ratio, or relative risk can then be calculated for possible causes.

9.4 Risk ratio and attributable risk

Cohort studies can provide the incidence ratio that compares the incidence for the exposed against the not-exposed. Incidence may be measured either as a risk (cumulative incidence) or rate (incidence density). A high incidence ratio is a good indication of possible causality. This is called the odds ratio in case-control studies and incidence (risk or rate) ratio in cohort studies. Case-control studies give the odds ratio because good incidence data are often not available whereas such data are available in cohort studies for calculating the risk or rate ratio.

Attributable risk measures the proportion of the risk in the exposed individuals who subsequently do develop the outcome of interest that can be attributed to particular exposures. There are several formulations for attributable risk, of which the most common is known as the aetiological fraction. This is often expressed as a percentage of the full risk that can be attributed to the particular exposures. For instance, about 90% of all lung cancers is often attributed to tobacco smoking.

9.5 Comparing case-control and cohort studies

Table 9.2 compares the advantages and disadvantages of case-control and cohort designs. This shows that the main advantages of a case-control design are for the study of rare diseases and to explore multiple possible causes. Cohort studies are particularly useful for detecting some rare causes, testing multiple causes, and identifying the average time period between exposure and disease onset.

Table 9.3 shows that the main methodological risks with case-control designs are high for both selection and recall bias, while for cohort designs the main risks are for loss to follow-up, the time period required, and the costs involved.

Table 9.2 Advantages and disadvantages of case-control and cohort studies

	Case-control	Cohort
1. Investigation of rare diseases or events	+++++	—
2. Detection of rare causes	—	+++++
3. Testing multiple effects of causes	—	+++++
4. Exploring multiple exposures and causes	++++	+++
5. Useful for long incubation periods	+++	+
6. Can explore time between exposure and disease	+	+++++
7. Measuring incidence	—	+++++

9.6 Regression analysis

The detected unadjusted associations may require **multivariate** analytical methods in which the health outcomes are studied in relation to more than just one or two possible explanatory variables. Multivariate linear regression can control for confounding caused by quantitative variables and regression analysis is useful when trying to understand confounding factors between several possible exposures (see Section 11.6).

Multivariate regression analyses help to assess whether an association between a possible exposure and the outcomes can be partially explained by a third or more confounding variables, such as socio-economic status. Logistic regression can be used when the health outcome variable is dichotomous (e.g. yes/no), such as individuals with or without diabetes. Although this analysis might suggest a possible cause, the strongest evidence for causality will come from experimental studies such as randomized controlled trials (RCTs).

Table 9.3 Methodological risks of case-control and cohort studies

	Case control	Cohort
1. Selection bias	high	low-medium
2. Recall bias	high	Low
3. Loss to follow-up	low	high
4. Confounding	medium	medium
5. Time required	medium	high
6. Costs	medium	high

9.7 Randomized controlled trials (RCTs) for efficacy

Controlled trials are particularly useful when testing a new intervention or a set of interventions for their ability to protect or treat individuals. There is a difference, however, between RCTs that examine the effects of interventions in individuals and the population effects of interventions in which whole communities are involved. The latter are often known as cluster-randomized trials.

An estimate of efficacy can be calculated when the intervention group is examined for a reduction in cases or an increased level of protection when compared to a control group. The risk ratios for participants in both groups can be compared and estimates of protection can then also be calculated.

Efficacy in individuals is usually estimated by RCTs (see Box 9.3). These trials provide the 'gold standard' for what different interventions can achieve when they are carried out under near-ideal and best circumstances. These trials are the most rigorous and best scientific way of testing the efficacy of new interventions. RCTs are an experiment where participants or groups of participants are randomly allocated to an intervention (treatment) group or to a control group. The results are assessed by looking for any significant difference between these groups.

These trials can, however, lack generalizability if the sample of participants is not representative of the people or patients in the specific population for whom the intervention is actually intended. Lack of generalizability can also be due to too many selected participants being declared ineligible or too many in the selected sample refusing to take part or are lost to follow-up.

There are usually three phases for RCTs, as, for example in vaccine trials. The first is the **Phase One Trial** or safety studies. These involve a relatively small number of volunteers being given the new intervention, and they are then kept

---

Box 9.3 Design of a randomized controlled trial

Time ⟹   - Intervention group   1. Disease outcome

Population - Random selection – Random   2. No disease
allocation

                         - Control group   1. Disease outcome

                                                     2. No disease

under close observation for any signs of adverse effects. If the proposed intervention then appears to be safe to administer and free from adverse side effects, the second level is a **Phase Two** trial that involves a larger sample of people to determine whether the intervention appears to produce the desired change or effect. For instance, a newly developed vaccine might first be administered to see if it appears to be safe at the injection site and for any other adverse reactions such as fever. If still found to be safe, then volunteers will be examined to see if the vaccine also produces new antibodies or an immune T-cell response as an indication of newly developed immunity.

The third is a **Phase Three trial** which tests the intervention for **efficacy** in people for whom it is later intended for, such as children, adults, and or the elderly. These trials test for the efficacy of an intervention or a set of interventions that might be used in patient clinical treatment protocols and in disease control programmes, such as for tuberculosis treatment, or the prevention of cardiovascular risk factors and their subsequent effect on heart diseases. Typically, Phase Three trials include many more participants than Phase One or Two trials.

Vaccine and other trials may include comparisons of a new intervention against a placebo as the control if there is no established prevention or treatment. Alternatively, a new intervention can be compared with a known and current standard for prevention or treatment.

A high efficacy for an intervention or set of interventions will lead to higher levels of cure or prevention when they are carried out in populations using the best quality guidelines and best practices. It is most important that efficacy is tested with people who are representative of the intended final target population group for the intervention(s). Interventions with high efficacy when implemented to the highest quality and with a high level of population coverage should result in a substantial reduction in the incidence of a disease or event or substantial improvements in levels of protection. With high efficacy such interventions should produce a given reduction in incidence, case-fatality rates, or case-disability rates or a higher level of protection.

When new interventions are implemented in the health services and public health programmes, it is important to have what are sometimes called **Phase Four follow-up studies** (these are not randomized trials) to monitor for:

- unintended side-effects which may only appear much later
- subsequent safety issues and previously unidentified side effects
- any reduction in the protection and benefits over time

Trials for efficacy can involve testing what level of protection or improvement is achieved by a single intervention like a vaccine or a new drug or by a package of evidence-based interventions like those for essential obstetric care, when a new vaccine is tested against an existing one or a new set of standard guidelines for antenatal care is compared to an earlier version. The results achieved with the new interventions are compared to those obtained in a control group of people who instead either receive the previous standard interventions or no interventions at all. In situations where it would be unethical to withhold treatment, such as chemotherapy for cancers, patients may be given the standard treatment together with the new drug to see if there is any additional effect.

Trials can also examine what improvements can be achieved when an exposure to a possible dangerous factor is removed. Such trials may be applied at the individual and community levels. For example, counselling individual smokers on stopping smoking or at community level when new environmental controls are implemented to lower the level of air pollution. For instance, what is the protective effect of introducing reductions in the levels of atmospheric particulates or nitrous oxide on the incidence of asthma attacks or when investigating the effects of restricting alcohol sales on indicators of mental health?

These trials can also estimate the full benefits of reducing or removing harmful substances all together. These trials usually require comparing communities rather than individuals—for example pollution controls will be enforced in some cities but not in others, which might constitute the comparative or control group.

9.8   Trials for community effectiveness

Effectiveness studies reveal what intervention programmes can actually achieve when routinely implemented to a high level of quality and coverage. Typically, the effect in whole communities is compared with the effects in control communities that did not receive the interventions. These trials measure the effectiveness of specific interventions, procedures, regimens, or services when they are delivered in ordinary and in real-life programmes.

Ideally, effectiveness studies are preceded by RCT efficacy trials such as when a new vaccine that was shown to be efficacious in a Phase Three RCT is rolled out through an immunization campaign, and researchers want to know the impact of the programme in terms of increased protection or a reduction in disease incidence in the whole population. These **effectiveness** studies are justified by the fact that administration of the vaccine or another intervention under routine conditions may differ from its administration under ideal RCT conditions. For example, the vaccine may not be adequately refrigerated, the injection technique may be faulty, or population coverage may be low and too many individuals at high risk of the disease may fail to receive the vaccine. For example see Box 15.2 on the effectiveness of a poor-quality measles immunization programme.

Effectiveness studies measure what is actually achieved when the interventions are delivered to the general population. They are also useful for identifying system bottlenecks to programmes that can reduce the impact of vaccines. Quality management should attempt to raise the level of effectiveness as close as possible to that for efficacy by performing according to the best quality management standards and guidelines. The aim is to reduce the gap between what could be achieved according to efficacy and what is actually being achieved by the more routine services.

Community effectiveness is quality × coverage × efficacy. For instance, what is achieved when new quality guidelines for tuberculosis control are introduced or a programme to reduce risk factors for obesity is implemented over a sufficient time period of five years? The effect of low population coverage on the effectiveness of immunization programme is illustrated in Box 14.4. This demonstrates the importance of achieving high population coverage.

The aim is to examine the effectiveness of interventions, either single or multiple, when they are delivered through public health programmes for whole communities. To achieve an impact, this requires that the new intervention or set of interventions is well implemented in the intervention arm for the whole community and in particular over a long enough period of time. It is important that the population intervention(s) is (are) delivered with satisfactory access to the interventions and that a high quality and good coverage are also achieved. New programmes may need one to two years to become fully implemented and a further period of three to five years before an evaluation is carried out.

Community effectiveness is often assessed through designs known as quasi-experimental studies, such as Before-and-After and Side-by-Side designs. These are not as rigorous as RCTs but they are often used in evaluation studies of population-based services and programmes. They can suffer from several methodological weaknesses, particularly with the controls and with confounding by external factors.

In the **Before-and-After** design (see Box 9.4), the control is what happened before in the same population compared to what is achieved after the interventions have been fully implemented, say for a further three to five years. This assumes that several years are needed to get the interventions fully implemented.

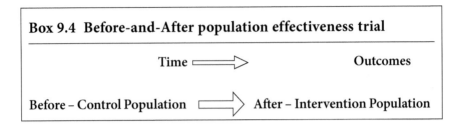

Box 9.4 Before-and-After population effectiveness trial

Time ⟹   Outcomes

Before – Control Population ⟹ After – Intervention Population

In the second **Side-by-Side** design (see Box 9.5) two or more similar populations are monitored over the same time period, say for three to five years, and the designated outcomes in the intervention and control populations are then compared over the same time period.

Both the Before-and-After and Side-by-Side designs can also be combined to provide a stronger design to measure outcomes. They can also both be used to examine long-term trends in data reported by the routinely reported health system. Baseline data are essential in both designs when the research needs to establish the prevalence or incidence of the disease before the introduction of the new intervention(s) and again to compare outcomes at the end of, say, a further five-year period of implementation.

9.9 Evaluation of public health programmes

Although both the previous designs are widely used to examine the effectiveness of public health programmes, both can also give misleading and faulty results if the methods are poorly designed and performed. In both designs it can be difficult to take into account in the analysis other widespread changes that are also happening in the local areas at the same time, such as changes in population age-sex structure, socio-economic developments, improvements in literacy, or dissemination of public media messages about health.

Box 9.5 Side-by-Side population effectiveness trial

Time ⟹   Outcomes

Intervention Population(s)

Control Population

In an attempt to control for societal changes occurring over time, one or more areas with the new interventions can be compared in a Side-by-Side design to similar control areas where the new intervention is not being implemented. However, different changes may still be happening in both the intervention and control districts. Some changes can be controlled for with regression analysis if the necessary data are available.

Governments sometimes designate that a new set or package of interventions, such as for a child health programme, be implemented in some districts and only later are they introduced into other districts. Community effectiveness and other indicators can then be used to evaluate an intervention district compared to other local control areas or districts or even with what is being achieved by other districts elsewhere in the country.

An advantage of this Side-by-Side geographical approach is that the government can organize a rolling programme involving new districts over several years, and the programme's success can be monitored for individual districts using estimates of community effectiveness as well as for the programme as a whole. This approach is sometimes called a **community stepped-wedge trial**. When the order of rolling out the intervention in different districts is randomly determined, stepped-wedge trials can provide more robust evidence of effectiveness.

An example of a trial to evaluate the effectiveness of a new package of child care interventions promoted by the World Health Organization (WHO)— Integrated Management of Childhood Illnesses (IMCI)—was carried out in several countries (see Box 15.3).

Many of these issues are considered further in Chapters 14 on health planning and management and Chapter 15 on monitoring and evaluation.

9.10 Ethics for health and research studies

Internationally approved guidelines exist for the conduct and organization of research and intervention studies, including the best ethical practices and the rights of the participants involved to be fully informed. More information is available from websites.

Phase One, Two, and Three trials all involve individuals who are volunteers and who are free to give their informed consent and who are also free to withdraw and refuse to participate. Consent is essential for all participants. The interventions must be delivered to the highest ethical standards, and all intended outcomes and all possible risks must be fully explained and declared to the participants before they enter into the trial. Protocols and trial methodologies also need to be submitted for full ethical and scientific scrutiny, including clearance and approval by a recognized research ethics committee (see Annex Five).

Ideally, trials also have an external advisory committee that monitors for safety and efficacy over time. When there are poor levels of safety or a high level of efficacy is achieved, the advisory committee may recommend stopping the trial as its continuation would be unethical in either case.

While routine health procedures in health services may not require such a review, research studies involving patients or the general population do require full ethical review and approval by a national Research Ethics Committee (REC) before research can start. This committee is often organized by the ministry of health, medical research council, or a national university.

Research involving local populations will need formal clearance and written approval by an REC. More details on ethical review are available in Annex Five and from research council websites. Most countries have procedures and committees to review the ethics of all health research proposals.

10

Organizing Investigations and Surveys

10.1 Using portable devices

Hand-held Portable Devices (HPDs), such as smart mobile phones and tablets, are now widely used in health investigations and surveys. They can be used for questionnaire interviews, sending data and messages, and for taking photographs and recording short videos. They can be used to facilitate contacts between health workers and patients, to disseminate clinic schedules, and to help maintain direct contact with households. Social media can also be used to distribute health messages using posters, pictures, and videos. It can also be used to encourage discussion and dialogue between health workers and community members (see Figure 10.1).

Survey questionnaires are now frequently installed on portable devices and data can be sent directly via the Internet to the survey headquarters for storage and analysis. These devices are also now frequently used for recording interviews, establishing geographic coordinates of households, ensuring that interviewers have actually visited particular houses, and taking photos of patient records and documents.

Interviewers ask questions and record the required information directly using Apps to code data on the device. Data entry checks are usually included in the device's programme so as to facilitate immediate data checking and processing after the coding boxes have been filled in and clicked. Consistency checks can also be built into the system and the data can then be sent directly via the Internet.

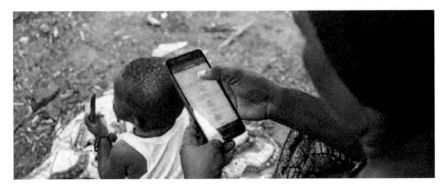

Figure 10.1 Communications using mobile smartphones

Data analysis programs allow for checking the entered data and if necessary for recoding the names of variables, which is useful when data are presented descriptively rather than by a numerical code and for when two or more files are merged. Checks on selected codes can be built into the HPD programme.

If paper questionnaires are used, both data coding and entry may have to be double entered or checked by another person to make sure it is correct. Mistakes can also be made in transferring pre-coded information to the appropriate coding box in portable devices. All coding and entry errors must be corrected before analysis starts.

10.2 Record forms and questionnaires

Two types of record forms and questionnaires are commonly used to collect information: one is given to the respondents to complete by themselves and is called a **self-administered questionnaire**. The usefulness of this approach largely depends on the complexity of the information required and on the literacy and honesty of respondents.

The second type requires an interviewer to ask for the information and it is called an **interviewer-administered questionnaire**. When accuracy and consistency are important, surveys and studies frequently rely on interviewers rather than self-administered questionnaires. Interviewer-administered questionnaires can be administered either face-to-face or remotely by telephone.

It is important that all information for one individual is collected together in one record form. This can be compiled from different sources to produce the epidemiological information, including from clinic registers (e.g. out-patient and mother and child health clinics), notes of patients under treatment (e.g.

tuberculosis and hypertension), records of special investigations undertaken (e.g. chest X-rays, blood examinations), or special registers (e.g. registries for cancer, congenital abnormalities). This approach is often used for special surveys and investigations.

A unique **identification number** for every individual in the survey is very important. If the sample size is less than 100, the individuals may be numbered from 01 to 99. The number can be more complex in a large household survey. For instance, in randomly selected clusters of villages, it may be necessary to identify persons by their village, house, and household by using a series of codes.

1	2 3 4	5	6 7
Village	House	Household	Person

For instance, the serial number 3-126-2-08 refers to the eighth person in the second household of house number 126 in village 3.

Unique identifiers are useful for tracing individuals and non-attenders and when the analysis requires respondents to be grouped together and when merging data files based on given criteria.

IDENTIFICATION NUMBERS HELP TRACK PEOPLE AND ANALYSE DATA

Questionnaires and record formats for individuals often contain five main kinds of data:

1. Background information, including names, ages, gender, and addresses
2. Household data, socio-economic status, and environmental information
3. Questionnaire-specific information
4. Results of physical, medical, mental health, and laboratory examinations
5. Additional data from laboratories and special investigations

10.3 Design of record forms and questionnaires

Formats must be carefully planned and pilot-tested. An example of a paper record form is included in Figure 10.2 and an HPD screen format in Figure 10.3.

COMMUNITY HEALTH SURVEY OF VILLAGE S (PERIOD: 1 April to 30 April 2020)

Date of interview: ___/___/___   Interviewer: _____

INSTRUCTIONS: 1. Fill in all the blank spaces, 2) Circle the appropriate answer in sections EH

Answer all items of information — do not omit any
Only fill in the boxes in the coding column if instructed

Coding column

Village: _____ (1)   House no: _____ (2,3,4)   ☐ ☐ ☐ ☐
                                                                       1 2 3 4

Household no: _____ (5)   Individual no: _____ (6,7)   ☐ ☐ ☐
                                                                       5 6 7

PERSONAL PARTICULARS

A *Name:* _____

B *Address:* _____

C *Sex:*   1 Male   2 Female   ☐
                                                                 8

D Date of birth: ____/____/____
                         Day Month Year

   Age last birthday (calculated from date of birth):_____   ☐ ☐
                                                                        9 10

E Present marital   1 Not married   2 Married   3 Widowed
   status: 4 Divorced/separated
                       5 Other (specify)_____   ☐
                       9 Did not answer/not known _____   11

F Ethnic group: 1 Malay   2 Chinese   3 Indian/Pakistani/Bangladeshi
                      4 African   5 Caribbean
                      6 Other (specify)_____   ☐
                      9 Did not answer/not known _____   12

G Place of birth: 1 Malaysia   2 Singapore   3 Indonesia
                      4 China   5 India/Pakistan/Bangladesh
                      6 Africa   7 Caribbean
                      8 Other (specify)_____   ☐
                      9 Did not answer/not known _____   13
                                           14
H Religion: 1 None   2 Islam   3 Christianity
                      4 Ancestral 5 Buddhism   6 Hinduism
                      7 Other (specify)_____   ☐
                      9 Did not answer/not known _____   14

Figure 10.2 Example of the first page of a pre-coded paper questionnaire form

Pre-coded answers facilitate data entry using a numerical value for each specific item of information and numerical codes facilitate data entry on portable devices. A category labelled 'others' is always useful for answers that do not fit into one of the pre-coded categories. The interviewer should specify these 'other' answers so that they can later be reviewed, coded, and analysed separately. Always include an option for 'not known' rather than leaving a question blank.

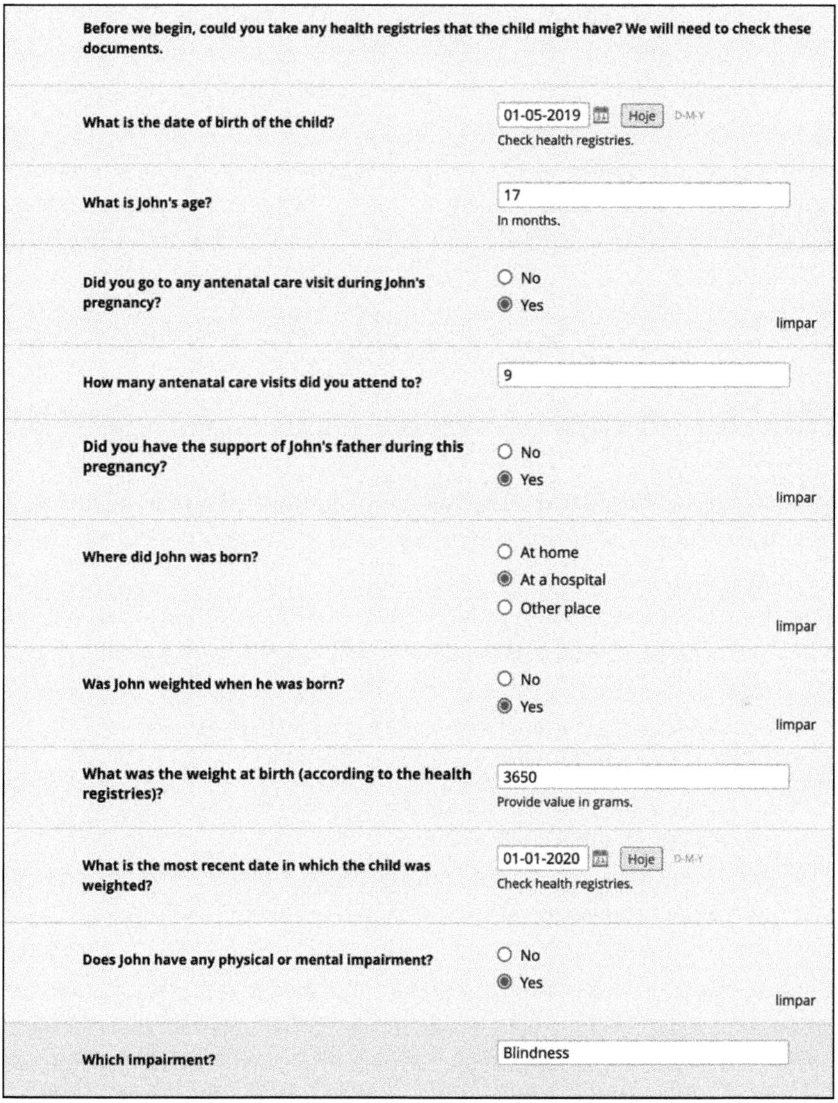

Before we begin, could you take any health registries that the child might have? We will need to check these documents.

What is the date of birth of the child?	01-05-2019 📅 [Hoje] D-M-Y Check health registries.
What is John's age?	17 In months.
Did you go to any antenatal care visit during John's pregnancy?	○ No ◉ Yes limpar
How many antenatal care visits did you attend to?	9
Did you have the support of John's father during this pregnancy?	○ No ◉ Yes limpar
Where did John was born?	○ At home ◉ At a hospital ○ Other place limpar
Was John weighted when he was born?	○ No ◉ Yes limpar
What was the weight at birth (according to the health registries)?	3650 Provide value in grams.
What is the most recent date in which the child was weighted?	01-01-2020 📅 [Hoje] D-M-Y Check health registries.
Does John have any physical or mental impairment?	○ No ◉ Yes limpar
Which impairment?	Blindness

Figure 10.3 Screen-print of an electronic child health questionnaire on an HPD
Courtesy of International Center for Equity in Health (Pelotas) www.equidade.org

The following guidelines apply to most data collection formats:

- Be suitable for HPDs and smart-phones
- Include a section for informed consent by all individuals
- Specify required individual data to facilitate entry
- Contain all the required information on the one form

- Be easy to use and with all sections in a logical sequence
- Should facilitate sending data for processing and further analysis

Interviewers should be adequately trained to use the questionnaire and their instructions, particularly if they are working on their own and far away from supervisors. Clear instructions help to avoid coding problems and it is better to spend more time training than have problems with data handling later.

ONE INDIVIDUAL PER FORM AND ALL INFORMATION ON ONE FORM

Guidelines on designing of record forms and questionnaires include:

- Interviewers need to establish a close rapport with the respondent
- Do not waste time collecting information that has little relevance to the objectives
- Avoid long forms and too many questions, which can annoy respondents
- Start with easier questions and save the difficult or embarrassing ones for the end
- Use clear and simple language written in a positive manner
- Avoid technical or ambiguous terms if possible
- Phrase questions in a conversational way and make sure that respondents can answer the questions
- Do not ask questions that are outside the respondent's experience or that occurred too long ago

Coding exact age needs a two-digit code. For instance, a 75-year-old man must be coded 75 and a 6-year-old girl would be 06. Coding exact individual ages makes analysis more flexible. Ages can also be grouped into 5-year intervals such as 0–4, 5–9, 10–14, 15–19, and so on. The age group 10–14 years, for example, comprises all children from 10 years to just below 15 years old. Children less than 1 year old (infants) are usually grouped separately from the 1–4 year olds. Larger age intervals can be used such as 15–44 years for females in the reproductive age interval, and 65+ years for older people.

Example: 'Where do you get your water from?' This might be coded as follows:

1 - tap in house	6 - spring, river, or lake
2 - tap or pump in yard	7 - other sources—specify
3 - tap or pump in public place	8 - not used for a code, or 'refuses to reply'
4 - open well	9 - Not known
5 - rainwater	

Example: 'How many living children do you have?' can be coded in two ways:

0__ None	5__ 5 children
1__ 1 child	6__ 6 children
2__ 2 children	7__ 7 children
3__ 3 children	8__ 8 or more children
4__ 4 children	9__ Unknown

Number of live children (circle):

0 (none) 1   2   3   4   5   6   7   8 or more 9 (unknown).

10.4 Planning investigations and surveys

Planning can be complicated and often requires more preparation time than expected. Survey objectives may have to be reviewed if they are too ambitious and the methods may require changes, such as a reduction in sample size, omission of particular questions, or fewer clinical and laboratory procedures. A pilot trial is essential to test the methods and planning.

Figure 10.4 gives an outline of some necessary preliminary steps and Figure 10.5 provides an example of a timetable.

A PILOT TRIAL IS ESSENTIAL FOR ALL METHODS, STAFF, AND EQUIPMENT

Is it necessary to change the survey objectives or scope?	Consider modifying objectives and scope of proposed investigations or survey	• Objectives • Methods • Location • Population • Time
Can resources be borrowed or obtained from elsewhere?	Consider availability of financial resources Are they sufficient for the study? Further logistics planning	• Staff • Materials • Equipment • Time • Money
Need for back-up plans and logistics	Use planning checklists	Consider all that is needed to organize and carry out the survey

Figure 10.4 Preliminary steps in organizing epidemiological investigations

	January	February	March
Weeks	1 2 3	4 5 6 7 8	9 10 11 12
Preparation - sample, forms and questionnaires	2 wks		
Recruit staff and obtain equipment	2 wks		
Pilot test methods and equipment	1 wk		
Train staff	1 wk		
Fieldwork		2 wks	
Analysis		2 wks	
Consultation on findings			2 wks
Final writing and distribution of report			2 wks
Total time required			**10–12 weeks**

Figure 10.5 Example of organizational plan and timetable for proposed survey

The following items need careful consideration:

- Approval—ethical approval and clearance, district governance, community acceptance
- Personnel—number of workers and different skills required
- Materials—records, questionnaires, equipment, laboratory tests, HPDs
- Finance—budgets for purchases, data analysis, fieldwork, allowances
- Time—preliminary organization, training, fieldwork, analysis
- Transport—vehicles, bicycles, and fuel

Obtaining approval has several aspects. If the survey or investigation is an integral part of delivering local health services or programmes, it may only be necessary to obtain managerial approval rather than formal ethical approval and clearance. This formal approval and clearance will be required, however, when research studies are undertaken by independent research institutes. It is essential that ethical principles are strictly adhered to for informed consent and confidentiality. See Annex Five for ethical review and clearance.

A chart can help with estimating the amount of time required to complete each stage (see Figure 10.5), which will indicate the total time required. Preparations and pilot-testing may overlap with training, but all three must be completed in time for the fieldwork. When preliminary consultations are complete it will be necessary to set dates well in advance for the actual fieldwork. All analysis and consultations should be completed before the final report is produced and disseminated.

If the survey or investigation involves people and their communities, it is best to discuss the plans with senior local government personnel first and to obtain the general consent of local community leaders. Consultation helps to strengthen public trust and encourages successful cooperation by the public.

The number and type of staff required depends on the necessary professional, technical and administrative duties. A task analysis of the survey may be needed before recruiting the correct staff if the survey is to be completed well and on time.

In some communities, women live secluded lives and men are not permitted to interview them nor enter their compounds or homes. Women in the sample may need to be interviewed by female staff, and sometimes husbands may answer questions for their wives and these answers may be misleading.

Materials depend on the survey and the amount required. Add extra for unforeseen developments and for any under-estimates. A budget is needed for such items as additional staff salaries, overnight allowances, accommodation, food and fuel, and for any new equipment, spares, or transport.

Although it is not usual practice in community studies to pay participants to attend interviews, something may be offered such as transport to and from the survey site or food as compensation for the people's time, particularly for those living in remote areas. Patients may need to be referred to the local hospital for a clinical illness or if they have missed out on any previous preventive procedures.

10.5 Organizing the fieldwork

If the survey or investigation involves a series of measurements on each attending participant, it is important to organize the work into separate stages that can be handled by different staff. Figure 10.6 shows an example for a nutritional survey of young children. To avoid confusion the sections on the record form should be in the same sequence as the different stations (numbered 1 to 7) and it is best if staff only obtain information or take measurements for their own section. Each interviewer/observer needs to sign their sections and forms to ensure their accountability and to make supervision easier when following up to correct any errors.

For household surveys it is important to be realistic about the number of interviews that an interviewer can safely complete in one day. Seeing the first respondents is easy but attempting to see non-responders requires much more staff time. Each household visit and interview may last 45–60 minutes and it is probably realistic for one interviewer to undertake only 5–7 household visits

Station 1	Registration and identification of individuals on sample list
(2 assistants)	and allocation of survey identification number
Station 2	Entering of name, address and other information on record forms,
(1 assistant)	questionnaires and labeling of specimen containers
Station 3	Interviewing patients or participants, assessment of age and
(2 assistants)	completion of health questionnaire
Station 4	Measurement of height, weight and arm circumference; eye test
(1 assistant)	
Station 5	Physical examination and recording of signs of malnutrition
(1 physician,1 nurse)	
Station 6	Specimens taken for laboratory tests
(1 assistant)	
Station 7	Clinic for any necessary treatments and medicines
(1 medical assistant)	Check the form is fully complete
	Thank you and goodbye. **Finish**

Figure 10.6 Example of an organizational plan for a nutritional survey

per day. Locating non-responders can be very time consuming which may reduce interviews to as few as one to three a day.

10.6 Logistics and support

For community surveys transporting staff and equipment (by road, water, or air) is usually essential and will require careful planning. Allow extra time for mishaps and pack all equipment carefully. If possible, arrange for back-up transport in case of emergencies. If necessary, make arrangements to transport subjects and participants to and from the different survey centres. Specimens may require special containers, labelling, cold storage, and transport, and a cold chain may be needed for biological reagents, specimens, drugs, and vaccines.

Good financial management is essential for staff morale. Salaries and allowances need to be paid on time and petty cash should be available for small local purchases. Keep a detailed record of expenditure and all receipts as the person in charge of finances may have to account for all funds spent.

In remote areas, local accommodation and cooking facilities may need arranging in advance and employing a site manager and cook can save on staff time. Food may require careful storage and bottled water may also be necessary, as well as facilities for refuse disposal and local toilets. As loss of stores and supplies due to damage and theft can be a problem, it is best to appoint one staff member as storekeeper so that they alone are in charge of issuing and storing any items.

10.7 Survey planning checklist

The following activities are listed in the order in which they might be performed

Planning

1. Decide why survey results are needed and how they will be used
2. Consult people with relevant local experience, including community leaders and health workers
3. Visit local areas to discuss the survey and for comments from the local leaders
4. Decide on objectives, necessary observations and measurements, and standardize the techniques
5. Choose an appropriate population sample
6. Design and pilot-test interview procedures, HPDs, record forms, and questionnaires
7. Make arrangements for ethical clearance, staff, equipment, transport, finance, accommodation, etc.

Organization

1. Obtain cooperation from local leaders
2. Train survey staff and their supervisors
3. Arrange for transport of laboratory specimens
4. Draw up a daily work plan for all staff
5. Pilot-test organizational details, including for staff, methods, and equipment

During the fieldwork

1. Supervise all staff closely to ensure high standards
2. Ask local leaders to help with organization and with attenders and locating non-responders
3. Make random checks on staff at survey centres and interviewers on their household visits

Analysis and communications

1. Analyse data as early as possible and perform checks daily
2. Discuss final results with health workers and community leaders for their comments
3. Write report, incorporate comments, and recommendations for new or improved health services
4. Distribute report and discuss recommendations with relevant local and national committees
5. Plan to evaluate any changes introduced as a result of the survey in order to estimate their effectiveness

11

Data Processing and Analysis

11.1 Data processing and analysis

Data only becomes useful information when they have been processed, analysed, and interpreted. Good quality data are essential and it can be unethical to use poor quality data. It is good practice, therefore, to ask some questions before analysing data, such as the following.

- How selective is the data collection? For example, relying on data collected only by health facilities can exclude people who are not using them. Data collection may have to be adjusted
- How accurate are the health data? Decisions based on poor quality and unrepresentative data may be unethical and might lead to unjust planning decisions and cost lives
- Is the data collection based on all people in the district population? For instance, are the poor, women, children, disabled, elderly, and ethnic minorities all fully represented? Unrepresentative data may hide inequalities and this may be ethically unacceptable
- How confidential and anonymous are the collected data? Household records and registers need to maintain confidentiality to protect the anonymity of individuals and disclosing names and addresses may breach confidentiality

Health data may come from different sources, such as **routine information systems**, surveillance, clinic records, epidemics, rapid assessments, and surveys and special studies. Processed data provide information on the most important **variables**. Analysis can be undertaken by hand if the sample size is less than 100 but using a computer is best for larger datasets. The first step is to check and clean the data. This helps immediately to correct any mis-recording and coding mistakes and it can also give a good 'feel' for what the data appear to be saying. After tallying it is then easier to calculate totals, percentages, and other summarizing statistics.

Computers can help with questionnaire design, data entry, and analysis. Health information systems in many countries rely on **hand-held portable devices** (HPDs) and computers at the local district level to handle health data, including for data entry and analysis. With appropriate computing software, statistical tasks are made easier, such as creating new variables or renaming them, grouping individuals, or selecting study subjects according to certain characteristics. A widely used programme is **EpiInfo** which can perform most routine analysis and statistical tests (see Section 11.9).

11.2 Summarizing statistics

Data on variables can often be expressed briefly by using **summary statistics** that are easily understood by local health teams. EpiInfo or similar programs can generate the following summary statistics:

- Percentages of subjects, for example schoolchildren with anaemia, malnutrition, or infected with malaria. A percentage is the number or ratio expressed as a fraction of 100 while a percentage point is the difference between two percentages. Percentages are absolute and percentage points are relative
- Proportion of subjects above or below certain cut-off points, for example systolic blood pressure of 140 mmHg or more for systolic hypertension and proportion of all pregnant women attending antenatal clinics
- Range showing the difference between the lowest and highest values in the raw dataset
- Mean or average, calculated by summing all individual values and dividing by their total number, for example mean birth weight, and average number of visits made by children to child health clinics

- Median is the value at the mid-point when the individual data are arranged sequentially from low to high. It can be used if data are skewed and do not have a normal distribution or where a few outliers would unduly affect the mean, such as very tall or heavy individuals
- Standard deviation (also shown as SD) can be used for data with a normal or bell-shaped distribution about the mean. A large SD indicates a wide scatter of individual values around the mean or average and a small SD indicates a narrower distribution. For example, child stunting is defined as children with more than two SDs below standard weight or length for age, and normal values for laboratory tests are often expressed as the mean plus or minus two SDs

The **p value** indicates the probability that the difference observed between two groups, such as men and women, could have occurred by chance alone, assuming that no true difference exists between these groups. This is known as the **null hypothesis.**

A p value of 0.05 or 5% is often used to reject the null hypothesis and that a statistical association probably exists between an exposure or intervention and the disease or outcome characteristic of interest. A p value of 0.05 means that the same result is only likely to occur by chance 1 in 20 times and a p value of 0.01 means once in 100 times. A chi square value of 3.8 has a p value of about 0.05. If a statistical association is found this does not mean there is a causal relationship.

DATA CAN BE PRESENTED USING SUMMARIZING STATISTICS

11.3 Steps in data analysis

Hand-tallying and sorting can be used by counting the number of times a particular piece of data appears in all the record forms by using a vertical tally mark and with the notation (////) used to indicate a group of five. This method can also be used for two-way and three-way tabulations, such as for mother's age and child's birth order.

Data for each variable or question are counted and the counts can then be summarized in tables that can be used to construct graphs, figures, and diagrams. All data must be classified into categories or numbers (e.g. haemoglobin values). Making frequency tabulations for each variable (or question), one at a time, is the first step in the analyses. Before starting the analyses, it is useful to prepare dummy tables based on the original objectives and the data to be collected.

Tables need to satisfy these conditions:

- All data must be classified into categories or numbers, such as spleen palpable (Yes or No), age (in years), or haemoglobin level (grouped or actual value)
- Categories must be mutually exclusive so that no individual can be classified twice in one table
- Each table must include all the 'raw' data
- No individuals can be excluded except in special circumstances and this should be noted
- Coding categories should include at least two levels and not more than ten as a general rule

Statistical analysis in epidemiology mainly starts by using three separate tabulations as follows:

- **Univariate** analyses, which include simple or one-way frequency tabulations, with each variable analysed separately; summary statistics such as means, percentages, and standard deviations may be calculated for univariate quantitative variables such as for height or blood cell counts
- To look for associations **bivariate** or **multivariate** analyses using two-way and three-way tabulations for two or three variables are used and summary statistics, such as means, percentages, and standard deviations may be calculated for each group and then compared, for example haemoglobin levels by age groups of children

11.4 Simple tabulations

Table 11.1 shows a set of raw data obtained from a cross-sectional prevalence survey of a random sample of 100 villagers for haemoglobin levels and hookworm infection, with additional information on the age and sex of the villagers. This data will be used to illustrate statistical tables.

If raw data is entered into a computer or handheld device using EpiInfo or a similar programme, the tables can be generated with the same software.

Table 11.1   Raw data for haemoglobin level and hookworm infection

Individual	Age (Years)	Sex	Haemoglobin (g/100 ml)	Hookworm infection
1	46	F	10.3	+
2	9	F	8.4	+
3	8	F	9.0	-
4	30	F	9.4	-
5	45	F	8.4	+
6	2	M	10.0	+
etc. up to 100				

The only difference from this table would be that the presence of hookworm infestation would have been coded on entry using either a No/Yes (N/Y) field or alternatively using (1 = No), and (2 = Yes). The sex can also be entered using (1 = Male) and (2 = Female). This numerical data can then be entered into the computer using EpiInfo and word labels can be added later.

Table 11.1 is based on a sample of 100 villagers identified by a census and with ten individuals selected randomly from each of ten randomly selected villages in the whole district, making a total sample of 100 individuals.

Simple analyses are limited and provide the first estimates of health status, such as mean levels of haemoglobin for the whole sample of individuals under study. These are referred to as univariate analyses.

In addition, it may be important to know if the health outcome, haemoglobin level, varies according to explanatory factors such as participant's sex, age, ethnicity, or socio-economic status. This requires bivariate analyses, for example, when the mean level or prevalence of the outcome is calculated separately for men and women. A statistical test for the p value is necessary to see if any differences may be due to chance—using the p level, as described above. This analysis is bivariate (two variables) and produces crude or unadjusted measures of the association between the explanatory variable and the outcome.

ANALYSIS STARTS WITH ONE-, TWO-, AND THREE-WAY TABLES

Table 11.2 shows the age distribution of the full sample of 100 villagers by broad age groups. This involves one discrete variable—age—in a univariate one-way table. Age is shown in broad age groups as the number of subjects is

Table 11.2 One way—age distribution of the sample of 100 villagers

Age group (years)	Number
0–4	19
5–14	25
15–44	40
45–64	14
65+	2
Total	100

Table 11.3 Two way—age and sex distribution of the sample of 100 villagers

Age group (years)	Male	Female	Total
0–4	10	9	19
5–14	12	13	25
15–44	20	20	40
45–64	6	8	14
65+	1	1	2
Total	49	51	100

fairly small, with only one child of 1 year old and one 71-year-old adult. Such a population is usually divided into between four and ten groups. For large samples, the number of age classes can be expanded using 5-year age groups, such as: under 1 year old, 1–4, 5–14, 15–24, 25–34, 35–44, 45–54, 55–64, and 65+ years.

Table 11.3 shows the age and sex distribution of the sample of 100 villagers according to a recent district census as a two-way table. The age and sex distributions of the sample can be compared to the whole population in the district. If the two are similar, the random sample is probably reasonably representative of the whole local population.

For a continuous variable, such as haemoglobin level, a simple tabulation can also start by grouping the data into categories, as shown in Table 11.4. The difference between the lowest and highest values gives the range which is 7.6 g/100 ml, the lowest being 6.2 and the highest 13.8. Intervals of one gram are often used.

Table 11.4 Distribution of haemoglobin levels
in 100 villagers

Haemoglobin level (g/100)	Number of villagers
6.0–6.9	5
7.0–7.9	6
8.0–8.9	13
9.0–9.9	22
10.0–10.9	29
11.0–11.9	14
12.0–12.9	9
13.0–13.9	2
Total	100

11.5 Cross-tabulations

Cross-tabulations involve two or more variables. The simplest form of a **cross-tabulation** is two rows and two columns. Table 11.5 is a two-by-two table which is often used when both variables are either 'present' or 'absent'.

The haemoglobin value of less than 10 g/100 ml is an arbitrary cut-off point for the diagnosis of anaemia, which affected 46 out of the 100 villagers and 59 villagers had hookworm infection, with 59.3% being anaemic compared with 26.8% for those with no hookworm infection.

A chi squared test is useful in 2 × 2 tables for statistical significance. This shows that anaemia was statistically associated with hookworm infection (p or probability < 0.05). Odds ratios and confidence intervals can be obtained using EpiInfo or another statistical software.

Table 11.6 shows a cross-tabulation for the two variables of haemoglobin and sex. To simplify the analysis the haemoglobin levels have been grouped into three categories (< 9, 9–10, > 10) and separately for males and females.

Table 11.7 shows a three-way tabulation with the three variables of haemoglobin and age groups in smaller categories and sex as male and female given separately in the raw dataset. One-way or two-way tables can be obtained from this three-way table by looking at the totals. For example, in the three-way tabulation given in Table 11.7, the row totals give the simple tabulation for haemoglobin levels.

Table 11.5 Distribution of hookworm-infected subjects and haemoglobin levels

Haemoglobin level	Hookworm infection			Hookworm (%)
	Present	Absent	Total	
Less than 10 g/100 ml	35	11	46	76.1
10 g/100 ml or more	24	30	54	44.4
Total	59	41	100	
% with anaemia	59.3%	26.8%		

Table 11.6 Distribution of 100 villagers by haemoglobin levels and sex

Haemoglobin level (g/100 ml)	Sex		Total (both sexes)
	Male	Females	
< 9	11	13	24
9–10	20	31	51
> = 11	18	7	25
Total	49	51	100

Table 11.7 Distribution of 100 villagers by haemoglobin level, age, and sex

Haemoglobin level (g/100 ml)	Age group (years)					Total
	0–4	5–14	15–44	45–64	65+	
	M F	M F	M F	M F	M F	M F
6.0	0 0	0 1	1 1	0 1	1 0	2 3
7.0	1 1	1 1	0 0	1 1	0 0	3 3
8.0	1 3	1 1	2 0	2 3	0 0	6 7
9.0	4 2	2 3	3 5	1 1	0 1	10 12
10.0	2 2	5 5	2 10	1 2	0 0	10 19
11.0	0 1	1 2	8 2	0 0	0 0	9 5
12.0	0 0	2 0	4 2	1 0	0 0	7 2
13.0	2 0	0 0	0 0	0 0	0 0	2 0
Total	10 9	12 13	20 20	6 8	1 1	49 51

11.6 Multivariate regression analyses

Simple survey analyses start with univariate analysis and then use bivariate analysis with two variables. These produce crude or unadjusted measures of any association, say between haemoglobin level and hookworm infection. However, there may be more than two variables involved. More complex analysis may require multivariate methods in which the health outcomes are studied in relation to more than one or two possible explanatory variables.

Regression analysis can be used to help understand **confounding variables**. For example, are children with many siblings more likely to be stunted or too short for their age? Is a large number of siblings associated with stunting? Are there other characteristics or confounding variables for these children that can explain this difference?

Multivariate regression analysis helps to assess whether the association between number of siblings and stunting can be explained by a third variable, such as the socio-economic status of the family. This third variable is referred to as a possible 'confounding' factor. Multivariable regression methods can adjust for socio-economic status in the association between siblings and stunting and the adjusted measure of this association can then be compared with the crude or unadjusted measures. If the association disappears after adjustment for a confounding variable, then it is likely that differences in socio-economic status account partially or in full for the apparent effect that the number of siblings is associated with stunting.

Multivariate analyses can be performed by EpiInfo which can perform linear regression for quantitative variables, such as haemoglobin levels. The **logistic regression** command is similar and is used when the health outcome variable is dichotomous (e.g. yes/no), such as individuals with or without diabetes. It can also perform Kaplan–Meier (KM) survival analysis which compares groups of individuals, such as for how long they remain alive after the diagnosis of a severe illness. A similar command is COXPH (Cox Proportional Hazards survival analysis) which also compares the survival of different groups of individuals.

Although this analysis might suggest a possible cause, the strongest evidence of causality will come from health studies, such as cohort studies and randomized controlled trials (RCTs).

11.7 Correlation for associations

Two quantitative variables are positively associated or correlated with each other when they either increase together, or when an increase in one is associated with a decrease in the other. If a decrease in one is associated with an increase in the other there is a negative correlation. For example, birth weight is positively correlated with mother's weight and the proportion of children with low weight-for-age is often negatively correlated with family income.

The **scattergram** is useful way to display an association when there are two continuous variables, as shown in Figure 12.12. The closer the mass of dots are to a straight line the more closely the two variables are correlated.

Correlation values can be calculated using statistical formulae and expressed as a **correlation coefficient**, which varies between –1 and +1. A coefficient close to 0 implies there is little or no statistical correlation between the two variables. Usually values below an absolute of 0.5, whether negative or positive, are not usually considered strong enough and they could have been due to random error. Values above 0.5 in either a–1 or +1 direction can be evidence for an association. Statistical software can generate correlation coefficients and show if this is statistically significant or not.

When two variables are correlated this does not necessarily mean that one variable is a cause of the other. Great care is needed when interpreting any relationship between associated variables.

11.8 Standardization

To compare two groups who have differences in their population age/sex pyramids it is necessary to standardize for these differences. For example, this is necessary when comparing two different populations for the prevalence of hypertension or malnutrition in an area today with any data for ten years previously, or between disease prevalence rates today in two or more different districts or even with national data for the whole country.

To take into account any changes or differences in population structure use can be made of percentages or age- and sex-specific rates per 1,000 people. For example, in comparing say the 20% of male children aged 5–9 years who were stunted and suffering under-nutrition in 2010 with the equivalent of 10% in 2020 a statistical adjustment is necessary. This can be performed using **direct standardization**. The same applies when comparing local and national rates when they have been based on different population age- and sex-structures or pyramids (see Annex One).

See Box 11.1 on the use of direct age standardization for villages A and B with different prevalence rates for *Schistosomiasis mansoni*.

The rates are averaged by using weights in the distribution of a specified standard population. The standardized rate represents what the crude rate would have been in the study population if it had the same distribution as the standard population with respect to both age and sex.

It is also important to standardize for age and sex structure if the risk of death is unevenly distributed. For example, it would be invalid to directly compare the crude death rates (CDR) in two different districts if a higher percentage of children are living and dying in one of the districts. This is also true if the age structure differs for only one sex, such as for the number of births or the risk of cervical cancer in women. It is even dangerous to directly compare local rates in the same district for today with those of, say, 10 or 20 years ago.

Box 11.1 Example for age standardization: comparing prevalence rates in villages A and B

Two villages, endemic for schistosomiasis, each had a population of 500 people who were examined for the presence of *Schistosomiasis mansoni* eggs in faecal specimens. The two villages were thought to be similar for their total population, age range, and male to female sex ratio.

The overall prevalence rate for the total population in village A was found to be 50.4% and in village B it was 37.4%. The difference between the two rates = 50.4 – 37.4 = 4.2, *p* less than 0.01.

It was concluded that a true difference existed for schistosomiasis prevalence rates and that village A was more heavily infected than village B. However, while the total prevalence percentages appeared significantly different, all the age specific rates were found to be the same in both villages. If the age-specific rates had been used instead the conclusion would have been different.

In village A the 10–14 years age group had more people and this led to a higher prevalence rate for the total percentage. When the analysis was standardized for population differences in age structure, there was in-fact no difference between villages A and B. The original conclusion was wrong because it had not taken into account the different age structures in villages A and B.

More detail on using disease-specific rates and direct standardization is given in Annex One.

Age/sex standardization is based on using weighted averaging to remove differences when comparing two or more populations in their age or sex structure or any other important confounding variable. This method is used to adjust rates in order to avoid incorrect conclusions.

> ## TO COMPARE TWO OR MORE POPULATIONS USE STANDARDIZATION

Age and sex specific rates can also be used. These should be specific for men and women combined or separately and for specific age groups. The numerator and denominator must both refer to the same age- and sex-specific groups.

Epi Info™ 7 Menu

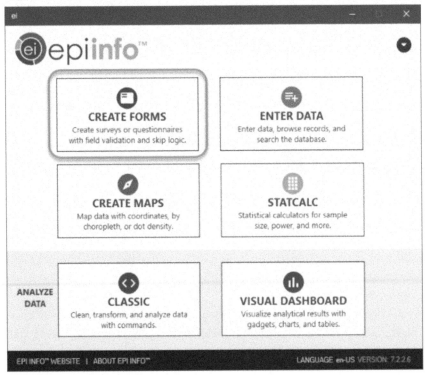

Figure 11.1 Using EpiInfo

Epi Info TM 7

Source: Epi Info™, Division of Health Informatics & Surveillance (DHIS), Center for Surveillance, Epidemiology & Laboratory Services (CSELS) CDC

11.9 Using EpiInfo

EpiInfo is a public domain set of software tools designed for public health practitioners and researchers. It is available in three versions: for Windows, for HDPs, and for web and cloud computing. Figure 11.1 shows the EpiInfo 7 menu for version 7 of the programme and provides an overview of its different functions and a user guide. <https://www.cdc.gov/epiinfo/support/userguide.html>

EpiInfo is a versatile programme and can be used for designing questionnaires, entering data, checking on data entry quality, and for data analysis (see Figure 11.1).

EpiInfo may also be used to calculate sample sizes needed in health surveys and studies. If data entry is performed by different people this can also be checked. Data can be exchanged between different software programmes using data import and export routines. If different files have been used in entering data, these can be merged into one file. It can also perform most routine statistical tests and create graphs and maps. It can analyse child anthropometric data and compare measurements with international growth standards and references.

Always protect and save entered data by keeping back-up duplicate copies on an external hard-drive or memory stick. Alternatively send attached files by email to yourself and/or use a cloud account. Back-up at the end of each day and lock computers away in a safe place. Remember to use passwords and/or PIN numbers for safety. Viruses can bring about loss of data and they can even enter a computer undetected when attached to an Internet e-mail or attached file. Using up-to-date antivirus software is essential.

12

Presenting Health Information

12.1 Tables and figures

Statistical tables are the main means for presenting analysed data, particularly numerical and quantitative data. Figures, graphs, and maps are also used to present visual information and show comparisons, patterns, and trends over time. Figures are also useful for showing qualitative or non-numerical information. Most statistical computer software can generate different presentations from tables to computer-assisted maps.

The following details are required and must be borne in mind:

- Titles should be self-explanatory, expressing all the information presented with a clear title: 'Prevalence rates by age for *Schistosoma haematobium* in five provinces of Zambia, July 2020'
- Rows and columns need to be clearly labelled and all categories clearly shown
- Axes of graphs and diagrams must be defined with scales that are clearly labelled
- The vertical axis is the Y-axis (ordinate) and horizontal axis is the X-axis (abscissa)

In Figure 12.1 birth order is on the horizontal axis, beginning with a value of 1 and increasing until the highest recorded birth order in the sample. The vertical axis shows the frequency of individuals in intervals of 10. The first bar

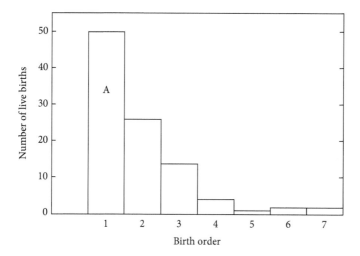

Figure 12.1 Distribution of 100 consecutive live births by birth order

Reproduced with permission from Vaughan, J Patrick, Morrow, Richard H, and World Health Organization, Manual of epidemiology for district health management, World Health Organization; Geneva, Switzerland, Copyright © 1989

(A) indicates that there were 50 infants of birth order 1 and the last three bars show only a few births. This is an asymmetrical distribution.

Keys or labels are necessary in graphs with more than one group. Labels identify the different groups being presented for comparison (see Figure 12.2). A diagram or chart may be reproduced from another source provided this is fully acknowledged with a footnote indicating the source.

12.2 Graphs

Frequency graphs: These show numerical data such as babies delivered each week, or new cases of pneumonia admitted to hospital per month, or percentages of children immunized by year. Figure 12.2 shows time trends for the number of different national health workers employed over ten years. The number of nurses almost doubled, from less than 3,000 to nearly 6,000, while midwives and doctors both only showed smaller increases. Graphs can also show *relative* change. For instance, pharmacists had the fastest increase with a threefold rise from about 100 to nearly 300 over the ten years.

Graphs are useful for showing time trends for two or more distributions providing the differences between the lines are clear. Figure 15.2 shows the

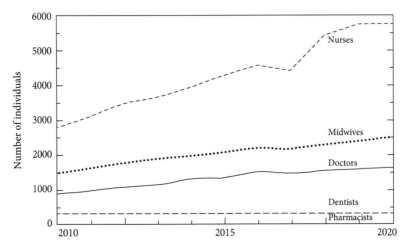

Figure 12.2 Growth in number of registered health workers, 2000–2010

Reproduced with permission from Vaughan, J Patrick, Morrow, Richard H, and World Health Organization, Manual of epidemiology for district health management, World Health Organization; Geneva, Switzerland, Copyright © 1989

number of mothers delivered each month in a district by trained traditional birth attendants (TBAs) during one year compared to the number delivered during the same period by professional midwives in the local health centres and hospitals.

Drawing a frequency graph:

- Draw the horizontal axis (X-axis) and mark the scale using equal units. Use the mid-point of each interval to represent all measurements in that interval
- Mark the vertical axis (Y-axis) to show frequency, usually as a number, percentage or rate
- For grouped data place mark where the vertical (frequency) and horizontal (scale) values intersect
- Join the marked points with straight lines that can be extended to the X-axis (see Figure 12.3)

Graphs can also compare two frequency distributions such as birth weight and sex. Figure 12.3 suggests there were more low birth weight girls than low birth weight boys.

Cumulative frequency graph: These can show progress in implementing a planned activity such as the total number of children of immunized (see

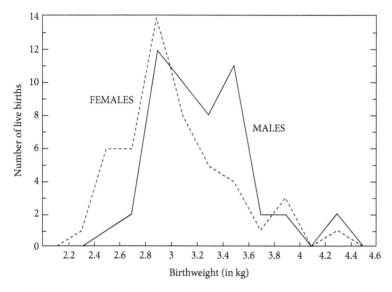

Figure 12.3 Frequency distribution of 100 live births by sex and birth weight

Reproduced with permission from Vaughan, J Patrick, Morrow, Richard H, and World Health Organization, Manual of epidemiology for district health management, World Health Organization; Geneva, Switzerland, Copyright © 1989

Figure 15.1). The frequency progressively increases, or if no further activities are added it remains constant over time and the graph line then flattens out.

Drawing a cumulative frequency graph:

- Add the number in each class of the distribution to the frequencies in all preceding classes
- For each class plot the cumulative frequency at the end of the class interval on the horizontal axis
- Join the points with straight lines to produce the cumulative frequency graph

12.3 Frequency histograms

These diagrams are commonly used and Figure 12.4 shows a typical example.

It is important that the bars of the histogram are joined with one bar immediately following another and with no space in between. The scale on the horizontal axis is a continuous measurement scale. This shows a bell-shaped

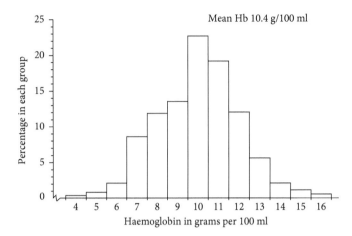

Figure 12.4 Histogram of the distribution of haemoglobin levels for 1,400 adult men and women

Reproduced with permission from Vaughan, J Patrick, Morrow, Richard H, and World Health Organization, Manual of epidemiology for district health management, World Health Organization; Geneva, Switzerland, Copyright © 1989

distribution and the standard deviation can be calculated for all the haemoglobin values. For a one-sided distribution (Figure 12.1) it is only valid to calculate the mode (see Section 12.1).

Drawing a frequency histogram

- The horizontal X-axis has a continuous scale with the vertical Y-axis showing frequency
- For each class draw a bar or rectangle. The width is the same value as the class interval used. The area of the bar should be the same value as the number of entries in that category. If the width of the bar is doubled the height of the bar should be halved

12.4 Bar charts

These resemble frequency histograms but the bars are separated by a space. This is used when the horizontal axis has non-continuous values or qualitative groups (see Figure 12.5). The variable or attribute is on the horizontal axis and the frequency on the vertical axis. Occasionally this is reversed. When percentages are used the sum of the heights of all bars should be equal to 100% (see Figure 12.6).

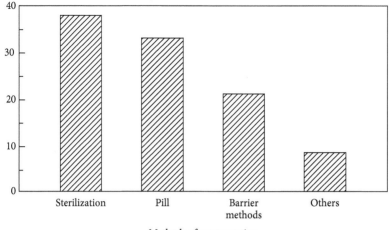

Figure 12.5 Bar chart of married couples practising contraception by main method used

Reproduced with permission from Vaughan, J Patrick, Morrow, Richard H, and World Health Organization, Manual of epidemiology for district health management, World Health Organization; Geneva, Switzerland, Copyright © 1989

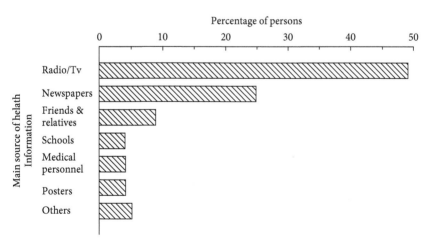

Figure 12.6 Bar chart of main sources of health information reported by a household survey

Reproduced with permission from Vaughan, J Patrick, Morrow, Richard H, and World Health Organization, Manual of epidemiology for district health management, World Health Organization; Geneva, Switzerland, Copyright © 1989

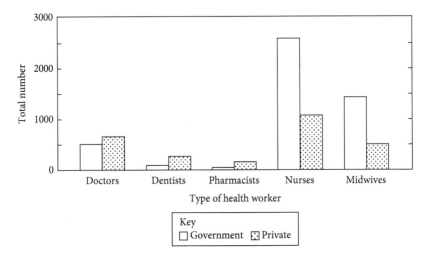

Figure 12.7 Multiple bar chart of health workers in government service and private practice

Reproduced with permission from Vaughan, J Patrick, Morrow, Richard H, and World Health Organization, Manual of epidemiology for district health management, World Health Organization; Geneva, Switzerland, Copyright © 1989

When comparing two or more distributions for descriptive variables, a multiple bar chart can be used (see Figure 12.7) to show, for example, the distribution of registered health workers in government service and those in private practice with each grouping represented by a pair of bars.

12.5 Pie charts

These circular and segmented diagrams represent the frequency distribution of a variable by groups or divisions and can also be used to compare two or more distributions. They are easily understood by people who are not used to handling numbers. They show percentage distributions so that a half represents 50%, a quarter 25%, and so on (see Figures 12.8 and 12.9). To draw pie charts it is preferable to use a computer programme.

12.6 Scatter diagrams

These are useful to display information on two connected variables that show a bivariate distribution, for example between birth weight and

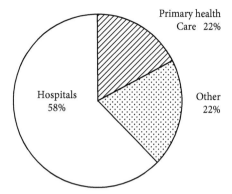

Figure 12.8 Percentage of health budget spent on hospitals and primary healthcare per year

Reproduced with permission from Vaughan, J Patrick, Morrow, Richard H, and World Health Organization, Manual of epidemiology for district health management, World Health Organization; Geneva, Switzerland, Copyright © 1989

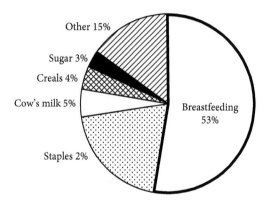

Figure 12.9 Main source of calories for infants aged 6–12 months

Reproduced with permission from Vaughan, J Patrick, Morrow, Richard H, and World Health Organization, Manual of epidemiology for district health management, World Health Organization; Geneva, Switzerland, Copyright © 1989

gestational age. A scatter diagram plots birth weight on the vertical axis and gestational age on the horizontal axis (Figure 12.10). The scatter shows each single individual represented by a pair of measurements. The dot in Figure 12.10 represents an infant with a gestational age of 35 weeks and a birth weight of 3 kg.

Scatter diagrams can reveal an **association or correlation** between the two variables, as in Figure 12.10, which shows a positive correlation between birth weight and gestational age. An infant with a high gestational age tends

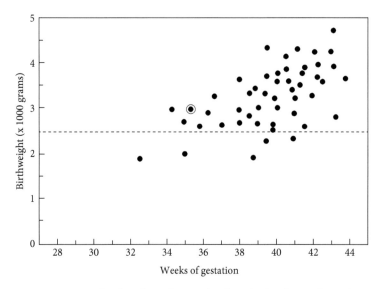

Figure 12.10 Scatter of 50 live-born hospital infants by birth weight and gestational age

Reproduced with permission from Vaughan, J Patrick, Morrow, Richard H, and World Health Organization, Manual of epidemiology for district health management, World Health Organization; Geneva, Switzerland, Copyright © 1989

to be heavier at birth than an infant with a lower gestational age. The diagram can only suggest a non-causal association and statistical techniques are necessary to measure and test its actual strength (see Section 11.7). Figure 12.10 also shows that 5 infants out of 50 had a low birth weight of below 2500 g, which is 10% of all births.

12.7 Maps

The value of detailed local maps is shown in Figure 12.11. During a review and analysis of hospital records it was found that most cases of onchocerciasis came from village A and some from B along the river, whereas most of the cases with *Schistosoma mansoni* infection lived in villages C and D, with some others coming from village B. A local environmental investigation showed that *Simulium* flies (the vector of onchocerciasis) were breeding in the main river, whereas the *Biomphalaria* snails (an intermediate host for schistosomiasis) were living in the creek. With such a detailed local knowledge of disease

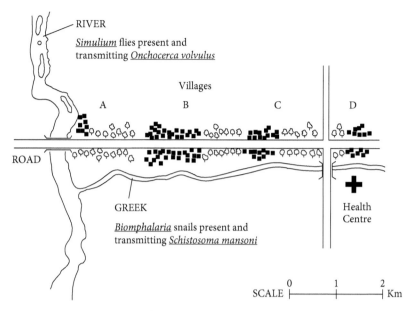

Figure 12.11 Transmission of *Onchocerca volvulus* and *Schistosoma mansoni* near four villages

Reproduced with permission from Vaughan, J Patrick, Morrow, Richard H, and World Health Organization, Manual of epidemiology for district health management, World Health Organization; Geneva, Switzerland, Copyright © 1989

transmission the control measures can be implemented more effectively at the appropriate sites.

Geographical positioning systems (GPS) have greatly improved the ease and accuracy of mapping and computer programs can draw district and regional maps. These are extremely valuable, particularly for showing the geographical distribution of the population and for the location of many different features, such as individual households, health facilities, protected wells and water sources, and roads and rivers (Figure 12.11 and Figure 15.3). They can also show the households where particular patients live, such as expectant pregnant women and tuberculosis cases under treatment. In an outbreak or epidemic maps are essential for showing the distribution of cases and their spread over time can suggest the disease itself.

Maps are essential for district planning and management, and central governments often publish maps for individual districts showing health facilities or comparisons between districts and for such health indicators as infant mortality rates or immunization coverage.

12.8 Photographs

Photographs are a powerful way of transmitting important information. It is simple to take photographs and videos with a mobile phone, such as for mosquito-breeding places near a school, a patient's clinic records, or patient's chart when attending an out-patient or mobile nutrition clinic. Photos of a patient's clinical condition can be forwarded for further consultation and advice. Photos are also a powerful means of sending information to higher level authorities for advice and corrective action.

12. 9 Displays on the district's performance

How well are the services and programmes improving? A display board in the district offices is another powerful way of documenting the progress of local plans. Charts, diagrams, and graphs, photographs can all be used to show how well services and programmes are performing for such operational indicators, such as percentage of deliveries by trained health workers, reductions in out-patient waiting times, or improvements in patient satisfaction following a reorganization of the hospital outpatients.

Examples might include improvements in drug availability, reductions in neonatal mortality following the introduction of a new standard delivery protocol, or guidelines for early infant care.

To show how the district is performing it is important to visually display figures, graphs, and photographs and these can also be forwarded to colleagues via the Internet. For instance, photographs can show plans and the location for a proposed new health centre, to display improvements in service quality, or to show the population coverage achieved by different programmes. This kind of visual information can be very convincing to staff by showing how programmes are performing.

13

Communicating Health Information

13.1 Importance of communications

Only analyse data if the findings are going to be used! Too often information from routine information systems, qualitative investigations, health surveys, or special studies is poorly disseminated and then often remains unused. Newly collected information must be used and communicated to local stakeholders and community members. What are the best communication strategies? These are best planned in the early stages of designing a survey or surveillance system. Local radio or television stations and social media platforms are important ways to communicate results and to pass health messages to the general public.

Health workers need to be familiar with their own local health information and use findings to improve health services and strengthen programmes. Findings, lessons, and recommendations can be included in local policy briefs, newsletters, and short written reports and shared with local health staff, discussed with community members, and shared with other districts, as well as with non-governmental organizations (NGOs) and the Ministry of Health (MOH). Also include other health-related sectors like agriculture, community development, education, water, and the environment.

It is important to inform local officials and other influential 'opinion leaders' of the results, such as teachers, health staff, and religious leaders. Also include community groups, local businesses, social and women's clubs, youth groups, and elected local representatives and officials.

> GOOD COMMUNICATIONS ARE VERY IMPORTANT AND USEFUL

13.2 Disseminating information

Social media

What are the most frequently used social media? Can important information be sent out as text messages? These platforms are useful to disseminate infographics, posters, pictures, and videos. A local team member should have responsibility to engage in dialogue with community members and media campaigns.

Mobile phones can send text messages, take photographs, and record short videos that can facilitate contacts between health workers and patients, disseminate clinic schedules, and maintain direct contact with households where patients live. Social media can also be used to distribute posters, pictures, and videos that encourage discussion and dialogue between health workers and local communities such as for TB control and maternal health programmes.

Policy briefs

These resemble newsletters and are used to disseminate information on local plans and strategies about new services and programmes, such as the reorganization of antenatal clinics or introduction of new service guidelines for diabetes or child care (see Figure 13.1). Graphs can be used to show the number of people attending clinics and coverage of different programme interventions. Videos can show health workers good and bad clinical practices and to use

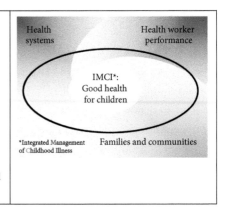

IMCI Strategy

Integrated Management of Childhood Illness (IMCI) is a strategy developed by the World Health Organization (WHO), Pan-American Health Organization (PAHO), and United Nations Children's Fund (UNICEF).

IMCI strategy aims to improve the health status of children. It includes three components: 1) improving case-management skills of health workers, 2) improving health systems support, and 3) improving family and community practices.

Health systems   Health worker performance

IMCI*:
Good health
for children

*Integrated Management   Families and communities
of Childhood Illness

Figure 13.1 Policy brief explaining the new IMCI strategy

with in-service staff training. Briefs can also help to encourage comments and identify barriers that different stakeholders have about local services.

Presentations to community groups

Personal communications with communities and key decision-makers can be very effective. These encourage public engagement through questions, discussion, and local involvement. They can be used to produce practical suggestions for local action (see Figure 13.2). Microsoft Powerpoint on a laptop is excellent for showing figures and photographs, and social media can be used to disseminate short videos.

Workshops

Dissemination workshops with key stakeholders are also a powerful way to convey findings and recommendations. Use flip charts, wall posters, and

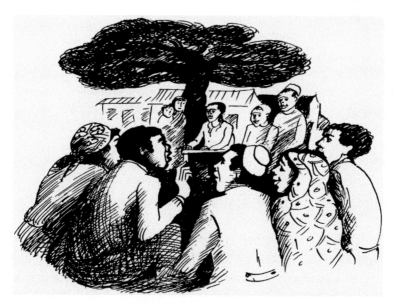

Figure 13.2 Discussing health information with community leaders
Reproduced with permission from Vaughan, J Patrick, Morrow, Richard H, and World Health Organization, Manual of epidemiology for district health management, World Health Organization; Geneva, Switzerland, Copyright © 1989

PowerPoint slides for graphs and figures. Workshops also provide opportunities to encourage discussion on possible solutions and next steps.

Posters and leaflets

It is best if these have a small number of key messages, such as 'Do not let your children die from malaria, take them to your health centre' or 'Diarrhoea kills through loss of water, use oral rehydration packets or ORS'. Posters can also be disseminated through social media.

Health education

Sessions can be organized when people attend health services and when mobile clinics visit local and village groups. Focus on appropriate priority messages and use questions and answers to encourage engagement. Avoid long didactic sessions. Health education teams can use campaigns for messages on immunization, latrines, or antenatal care. Publicity might involve churches, mosques, schools, and markets. Include information on days and times for meetings given out in advance.

Local radio and other media

Many countries have popular local radio networks and television channels that can broadcast important health messages. Health topics can also be included in popular local 'soaps'. Keep talks simple and avoid technical jargon. Practical messages can help people improve their own knowledge and lives.

13.3 Making presentations

Health managers may need to make presentations to meetings and to explain health plans to local leaders or community members and to present findings from rapid assessments or surveys to other public health professionals and planners in the MOH. Short videos can be disseminated through social media. The following can increase the effectiveness of such presentations.

Good preparation: Be clear on the main points to be communicated and keep the main messages short and simple. A short summary of main points can be distributed beforehand to encourage discussions.

Meeting place: Make sure that information has been sent out about the topic and time and place to meet. Arrange the seating and test microphones.

Projecting slides: Visual aids include flip charts and Powerpoint with an LCD projector. Effective slides are simple, clear, visible, and focus only on one or two main points. Use large letters that can be seen from the back of a large room. Avoid placing too much information on a slide and use key phrases and short sentences. Graphs are more effective than tables.

Practice speaking: Practice in front of colleagues and identify the points to emphasize and clarify.

Giving the presentation: Welcome the audience and briefly outline the main points. A golden rule is first say what you are going to say, then say it. Speak slowly, keep good eye contact, with the audience and speak facing them. Avoid looking too often at your notes and use a screen pointer.

Concluding the presentation: Repeat the main points in a brief summary. Leave the audience with 'take home messages', the most important points from the presentation you want them to remember and act upon. Thank them for their attention.

Things to avoid include: Poor preparation, talking too fast and too long, turning your back to the audience, unreadable slides, and making too many points in rapid succession.

13.4 Health reports

Well-written reports and briefing papers can be used to support local strategies and plans. These need to be both feasible and relevant to decision-makers. All reports should include an executive summary that conveys the key messages and use straightforward language with few technical terms. Distribute to all local key officials and stakeholders.

A well-written and detailed report is fundamental to communicating important local health information based on qualitative investigations, surveys, and special studies. Reports can carry a great deal of status.

The style and content of the written reports will depend on their nature and purpose as well as who is likely to read them. Consider the following points carefully:

- The title must clearly explain what the report is about
- Write clearly and use simple language with short sentences and paragraphs
- Consider who is the target audience and tailor the report to their level of understanding

- It should preferably only be about five pages and less than ten pages, with a good summary
- Main findings may be transformed into infographics
- Distribute through social media

It is best to discuss an early draft report with colleagues and community leaders before producing the final version. It may take several drafts before the final version is agreed.

A scientific paper or report usually contains the following sections which may be subdivided or combined, and items may be rearranged to make more appropriate sections.

Title page.   Full title of the report, names of the authors and their positions and addresses.

The title must be clear, for example 'Malaria in Amber District: the prevalence of *Plasmodium falciparum* infection in ten villages in July 2020'.

Executive summary.   Placed after the title page and limited to the main findings and recommendations. To retain the reader's attention this should not be more than 400 words.

Introduction.   This sets out the background information and purpose of the study and the reasons for carrying it out. Relevant literature and any previous work can be summarized and quoted here.

Objectives.   These must be clearly stated. For example:

'To measure the prevalence of *Plasmodium falciparum* infection in ten villages in Amber district during 2020' or 'To identify high-risk groups for obesity with regard to age, sex, and residence'.

Methods.   Describe the study population, sampling methods, selection of controls, and explain response and non-response rates and representativeness of the sample. Briefly describe all variables including age, sex, ethnic group and occupation, diagnostic criteria for diseases, and briefly explain procedures. These are important to judge methods and comparability of the findings to other studies.

Mention if a pilot survey was carried out and briefly describe the survey methods for collecting the data. A copy of the questionnaire or record format can be attached as an annex to the report. Describe interviewer training to minimize non-sampling errors due to variation and bias.

Results.   Include all the most relevant findings in the text and using tables, figures, and diagrams. For qualitative findings use illustrations and actual quotes from participants. Tables and figures must be self-explanatory and check that the table totals are correct. Label graphs clearly.

Discussion. Interpret the findings and make the conclusions clear. Include comparisons to any other relevant studies and state any obvious methodological limitations. Authors may give their own opinions here and can suggest explanations for the findings.

Recommendations. These should be listed and numbered, together with any suggested actions for disease control or improvements to public health programmes. Recommendations for improvements can include those for community organizations, local authorities, and the MOH.

References, acknowledgements, and appendices. Material that is not essential in the main report can be placed in annexes.

It is important to acknowledge all scientific advice and any donor support. Copies of the report should be sent to the ministry of health, donor organizations, development partners, and UN agencies.

13.5 Written reports

The length of a report will depend on the scope of the work, but the following is a guide. Since reports nearly always end up longer than originally intended it is best to aim for a maximum of ten pages.

	Number of pages Recommended	Maximum
Title page	1	1
Summary	0.5	1
Introduction	0.5	1–2
Methods	1–2	2–4
Results	1–2	3–4
Discussion	1	3–4
Recommendations	1	2
References	1	1
Suggested length	**6**	**10–15 (excluding title page)**

14

Epidemiology and Health Planning

14.1 National health plans

Epidemiology is essential for collecting and interpreting local health information and for producing local health plans. Epidemiological information is also crucial for guiding the local allocation and distribution of staff and resources, for monitoring implementation, and for the management of services and programmes. It is also essential to assess their access, quality, and coverage and to measure reductions in incidence of diseases and changes in health status over time.

A country's long-term development goals and health policies are usually the responsibility of the national government. Most countries have accepted primary health care (PHC) as one of their main health strategies to achieve the Sustainable Development Goals (SDGs) and to implement Universal Health Coverage (UHC). National health plans also take into account the country's particular health problems and the national resources available for health. Planners have the difficult task of working to improve the health status of whole populations while also aiming at the same time to reduce health inequalities between different population groups and diverse geographical areas.

The Ministry of Health (MOH) may state its long-term planning goals in broad terms such as:

- To maximize the total amount of healthy life for the population, and
- To ensure that everyone has access to high-quality and priority health services and programmes

To achieve these goals national health plans frequently set quantitative targets for the whole country. Targets are specific and quantified goals that are to be achieved over a specified time period, such as over five years. Examples might be:

- Infant mortality to be reduced from the national average of 60 to 40 per 1,000 live births per year
- Health facilities to be developed so that 80% of the population live within 10 km of a facility
- Supervised antenatal care and deliveries to be expanded from the current national coverage of 40% to at least 80% over the next ten years for the population living within 10 km of a facility or a trained health worker

With stated goals and time-bound targets, the MOH can then produce medium-term and five-year health plans for the whole country. These usually aim to combine strengthening the existing local primary health care services while at the same time also expanding the national promotive, preventive, and curative health services and programmes. In addition, plans will also be needed for the training and retraining of the health workforce. This includes strengthening the existing district health services and programmes as well as the allocation of financial resources needed to expand the district health system.

National health plans are the starting point for improving district health services and their local management. To develop the national plans the MOH will need substantial inputs from districts on health information and to decide on how to allocate the finances for recurrent and capital budgets equitably for the following years. Some governments have decentralized some of these financial responsibilities down to the regional or district level.

Rather than relying on fixed five-year planning cycles some countries rely on a system of rolling plans that cover three to five years ahead. Rolling plans focus mainly on detailed planning for the next one or two years and less detail for the following three years or so. Each year the detailed annual or biennial plans are agreed in more detail for the following one or two years and these are subsequently then rolled forward by one or two years. In this system the district's annual or biennial plans can be the most important ones.

Often national and district plans have to take into account the existence of significant differences and inequities between districts when compared to the national average. For example, in Bangladesh total fertility rates vary from 1.8 in Khulna District in the south to 3.7 in Sylhet District in the north. It is important, therefore, that planning takes into account such spatial differences in health status and does not just rely only on national statistics which are usually an average that hides wide variations between different districts.

14.2 District health plans

Responsibilities of local health teams are outlined in Chapter I and this chapter presents the use of epidemiology in district planning to strengthen primary health care. Local health planning depends on combining the guidance contained in the national plans together with local health information and local plans. However, details will depend on how local health services and public health programmes are actually organized in individual countries, including for the mix between government, non-government, and private services.
Health planning asks three important questions:

- Where do we want to be in the future?—'There'
- Where are we now?—'Here'
- How do we get from 'Here' to 'There?'

Where do we want to be?—This requires the development of national priorities for health policies, strategies, and plans, stated in operational terms, and with clear goals and targets to be achieved.

Where are we now?—This involves assessing the current health status of the local district population, identifying the number and range of national, local, and non-governmental health facilities, the number of trained staff, distribution of specialized services, availability of different equipment, and the budget allocations for recurrent and capital finances.

How do we get from here to there?—This involves determining how to tackle national and local priorities as well as how to organize the existing facilities at the same time while also planning to expand new health facilities and the training of new staff. Epidemiology helps to support and strengthen the local health management system. This planning sequence can be shown as a series of steps from national planning towards achieving local district impact, as follows:

- **Policies and priorities** formulated for national planning
- **Deliver** interventions as local clinical services and district public health programmes
- **Access** improved to locally delivered services and programmes

- **Quality** of services and programmes based on national guidelines/standards
- **Coverage** improved for high priority population-based programmes
- **Impact** achieved for disease reduction and for improvements in health status indicators

Epidemiological skills are crucial if the local health teams are to be successful. Local plans start with an analysis of the present national health plans and priorities that need to be tackled nationally and this is then combined with local knowledge of the districts and the involvement of local government, community organizations, and non-governmental agencies.

Strengthening of PHC for the SDGs and UHC depends, therefore, on national and local health plans working together with the available human and financial resources. The following are some commonly adopted national strategies:

- Decentralization by the MOH and strengthening of the local health systems
- Training of district health staff in planning and management
- Use of community health workers and other available human resources
- Community involvement to support local health services and programmes
- Collaboration and coordination between government and non-governmental agencies and services, as well as with private health facilities and practitioners
- Inter-sectoral cooperation with other health-related sectors, such as housing, water and sanitation, education, home affairs, industry, and agriculture

Local health teams need reliable health information and the necessary finances to set objectives for district services and programmes for the coming years. How well these are delivered depends on achieving improvements in delivery, access, quality, and coverage. Local planning must also take into account the existing staffing capacity to deliver any changes as well as taking into account equity and inequalities, community perspectives, and the public's trust in local services.

District planning for PHC includes reviewing the eight basic elements shown in Box 14.1. Some countries have expanded this list while others decide to give higher priority only to some of them.

It is also important for district teams to have a clear understanding of the available local health facilities, numbers of staff, and finances. If the population's health status is to be improved then priority should be given to

---

Box 14.1 Eight basic elements of primary health care

---

1. Treatment of common diseases and injuries for outpatients
2. Clinical care and investigations for inpatients
3. Public education on local health problems and their prevention and control
4. Promotion of proper nutrition and food supplies
5. Maternal and child health care, including family planning
6. Immunization against the major infectious diseases
7. Prevention and control of locally endemic and epidemic diseases
8. Promotion of safe water supplies, basic sanitation, and adequate housing

---

first improving delivery and access to the existing national services and programmes, and then second to improving their quality and coverage for the whole district population.

DO DISTRICTS HAVE MEDIUM- AND LONG-TERM
HEALTH PLANS?

14.3 Systems approach for services and programmes

A health systems approach to planning health services and public health programmes involves five interconnected stages, starting with planning the necessary inputs through to achieving impact as shown in Box 14.2.

Box 14.2 Systems approach to local health planning, monitoring, and evaluation

---

INPUTS	PROCESSES	OUTPUTS	OUTCOMES	IMPACTS
Plan	Organize	Deliver	Achieve	Evaluate

   Inputs—includes all the actions necessary to agree and start implementing the national and local health plans. This starts with a review of the national health policies and priorities, combined with local epidemiological information, distribution of local health facilities, numbers of different health workers, and availability of future recurrent and capital finances.

Processes—involves bringing together all the above components in order to organize and implement the local plan in the specified time period, including the intermediate and time-related goals and targets.

Outputs—includes early intermediate measures in the plan to build capacity and establish new health facilities, to deliver health interventions, and to strengthen existing curative services and programmes.

Outcomes—are intermediate measures of what the planned interventions aim to achieve. These are often used as proxy indicators towards reaching the required impact for changes in health status.

Impacts—involves evaluating changes in health status to reveal whether the plans have indeed achieved better health and led to positive (or may be negative) changes. Improving health status is a long-term objective as these changes only happen slowly and usually require strong programmes for many years.

The systems approach is equally useful when planning public health programmes that use evidence-based quality interventions to achieve improvements in the local population's health status. This requires that district health plans:

- **Deliver** essential services and programmes close to people's homes through health facilities, clinics, community health workers, mobile clinics, and outreach campaigns
- Improve **access** to essential services and programmes so that, for example, 80% of people have access to a health facility within 5 km or 10 km of their home
- Achieve **high-quality** health interventions that are conducted and delivered according to high evidence-based international standards
- And achieve high **coverage** of the total district populations at risk if health status is to improve

An example of the systems approach for immunization is given in Box 14.3.

Coverage is the most critical indicator for effective management. It shows what needs to be improved and who are the priority at-risk population groups. It also indicates what proportion of the target at-risk group are not receiving the interventions they need. Is the present distribution of interventions and services fair and equitable?

While coverage is the most critical indicator for effective management, it might be that the local health team may decide to give a higher priority to

184 EPIDEMIOLOGY AND HEALTH PLANNING

Box 14.3 Systems approach for child immunization programmes

Inputs (plan resources) include personnel trained to undertake vaccinations, vaccine doses, equipment for cold-chain and sterilization, needles and syringes, and records. Clinic rooms for sessions, waiting areas, and safe storage of equipment. Health education and community mobilization may be needed to encourage and increase attendances if too few mothers and children are attending.

Processes (organize activities) involve providing information and publicity about immunizations, looking after sterilizing equipment, arranging clinics, registering and screening children, conducting general health education with mothers, administering vaccines, recording immunizations, counselling of mothers on any side effects, and arranging dates for next attendances.

Outputs (deliver results) include the number and proportion of the targeted children receiving the various vaccines, vaccine doses used, and those wasted.

Outcomes (achieve coverage) is an increase in children fully immunized towards reaching 80% coverage of all children aged under one year old in the local population.

Impacts (evaluate improvements) is a reduction in morbidity and mortality from the disease(s) against which vaccinations are given, such as a reduction in measles incidence and mortality.

---

improving another service or programme while at the same time maintaining an existing programme at the same level over the following years.

The systems approach is also useful for public health programmes, as summarized in Table 14.1.

14.4 Current health situation

The starting point for local planning is the local health profile for the current health situation and the choice of indicators to measure progress towards the SDGs and UHC. This requires a good local knowledge of all the available

Table 14.1 Systems approach for selected public health programmes

INPUTS Plan resources	PROCESSES Organise	OUTPUTS Deliver	OUTCOMES Achieve	IMPACTS Evaluate
Family planning supplies, trained staff, and clinics	Family planning delivered and accessible	Regular users and more acceptors	Family spacing Fewer abortions	Lower fertility and birth rates
Maternal health antenatal/ delivery care guidelines	Clinics, medicines, trained staff, delivery	Safe deliveries, Newborn care Referrals	High quality and coverage	Reduced maternal mortality ratio, neonatal deaths
Child nutrition guidelines and trained workers	Nutrition clinics, education, rehabilitation	Breastfeeding and better-quality diets	More babies breastfed, less malnutrition	Improved infant nutrition and child growth
Child health guidelines for IMCI	Clinics, staff trained and supervised	Improved clinical care of sick children	Fewer deaths from diarrhoea and pneumonia	Lower infant and child-mortality rates
TB guidelines, staff, and drug supplies	Case detection, referrals, and treatment	Attendance monitored, cure, and resistance	Lower dropout, cases complete treatment	Higher cure rates, reduced incidence of new cases
NCDs hypertension and obesity guidelines	Education on diet, exercise, healthy behaviours	Reduced salt and calorie intake, more exercise	Risk behaviours changed, less obesity	Strokes and heart attacks prevented, normal weight

district health information, including on the population (Chapter 3) and local health data from the information system (Chapter 4). Keeping the district health profile up to date should be an annual activity and a display of indicators will be helpful in communicating progress.

Basic health status indicators often include nutritional status, fertility, morbidity and mortality, with resources indicators for facilities, staff, and administration. Minimum health services indicators are required for all clinical care services, and the public health programmes that are needed for pregnancy and delivery, childcare, environmental health, and communicable disease control. Many countries will have a similar or expanded list of basic indicators.

The local health profile has the following five main categories for data and indicators:

- Local population
- Health status

- Health resources
- Health services
- Health programmes

ANALYSE THE PRESENT SITUATION USING THE LOCAL
HEALTH PROFILE

14.5 Inequalities and local priorities

There is no single or 'right' way to tackle inequalities and decide on priorities and health interventions are required over a long period of time. For instance Figure 14.1 shows information on coverage and inequalities for the reproductive and maternal health programme interventions in Brazil from 1986 to 2013. Repeated large-scale surveys were needed to collect this information over many years

Policies can be chosen based on which ones will have the greatest impact on improving health status and reducing inequalities, or on lowering disease frequency, morbidity, and mortality, or even on evidence for the most effective and least costly interventions. People living in rural areas are often disadvantaged and left behind compared to those in urban areas.

Over a period of more than 25 years equity did improve in Brazil, with marked improvements in programme coverage and a reduction in inequalities. In 2013 the rural–urban differences were much smaller, which shows that if inequalities are to be reduced it is important that consistent support for health services and programmes is maintained over long periods of time. Much of the Brazilian improvements are explained by an expansion in access to family health programmes in rural areas and an expansion in hospital networks.

14.6 National and district planning

How to decide on which local health services and programmes need strengthening? National health plans list the country's national priorities and the important political, social, and economic factors involved in national decision-making. National priorities help local teams to identify and decide on their local priorities. This may also involve consulting with other local non-government providers, community representatives, local councils, and other government departments.

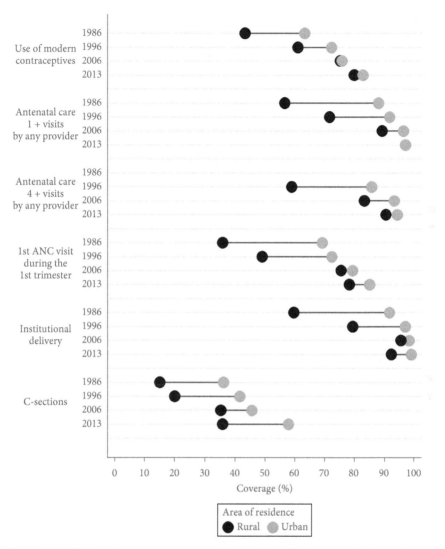

Figure 14.1 Information on coverage and inequalities for the reproductive and maternal health programme interventions in Brazil from 1986 to 2013

Reproduced from França, GV, Restrepo-Méndez, MC, Maia, MF, Victora, CG, and Barros, AJ (2016). Coverage and equity in reproductive and maternal health interventions in Brazil: impressive progress following the implementation of the Unified Health System. International Journal for Equity in Health, 15(1), 149. https://doi.org/10.1186/s12939-016-0445-2 with permission from Springer Nature
<https://creativecommons.org/licenses/by/4.0/>

Local plans include how to get from 'Here' to 'There'? This will include an analysis to support the following stages:

- Identify the priority local health problems, including for inequalities
- Define high-risk and disadvantaged groups of people
- Plan to improve the delivery of services and programmes
- Identify capacity and gaps in the delivery of services and programmes
- Improve access to health services and programmes
- Improve the quality of services and programmes
- Estimate the coverage of the existing health services and programmes
- Examine how adequate is the management and administration of all services and programmes

Deciding on priorities is important because local health resources are usually limited. For instance, what priority should be given to which services or programmes? Which population groups, health risks, diseases, or underlying health problems should have high priority? Which health programmes should receive more or fewer resources? Epidemiological health information helps to answer these questions.

> ## PLANNING INVOLVES DECIDING ON PRIORITIES AND MAKING DECISIONS

Epidemiological knowledge and experience are essential for deciding on priority diseases and on which underlying health risks and diseases should also be given priority. Priority is often given to diseases that are frequent, severe, and cause high morbidity and/or high mortality. Should other effective and cheaper interventions be considered? Another choice may have to be made between investing in priority programmes and developing new health services or facilities. Discussions on priorities can also be held with community representatives, government officers, private health service providers, and local NGOs.

District health plans also have to achieve a balance between the following broad priorities:

- Health policies to tackle inequalities, such as between urban and rural communities
- Health promotion and prevention programmes, such as health education, mother and childcare, immunization, nutrition, and environmental health

- Communicable diseases control programmes, such as for human immunodeficiency virus (HIV), tuberculosis (TB), malaria, and measles
- Non-communicable diseases (NCDs), such as for cardiovascular risk factors, hypertension, and diabetes
- Curative services for ill people, based on primary health care facilities and referrals to hospitals
- Improving people's access to these services via community health workers, health centres, and other outreach and mobile services
- Developing and upgrading of health worker skills through in-service and retraining programmes
- Management and administrative support, analysis of local information, and improving equipment, transport, and communications

Local epidemiological information can help the district team focus on common health problems although some uncommon communicable diseases, for example African trypanosomiasis and dengue fever, may have low frequency but are important because they can lead to severe epidemics.

Choices may also have to be made between improving access by building new facilities or expanding the capacity of existing services, or organizing and planning for new priority interventions. These choices may well be contentious and can be at risk from political interference.

14.7 High-risk groups

Another way to manage priorities is to consider which groups of people should receive priority in the district. People at higher risk of morbidity or mortality are called high-risk groups, such as the poor, marginal, and people who underutilize existing services or indeed may not even have access to the health care they need.

Epidemiological information is essential to define high-risk groups which can include:

- Reproductive women aged 15–44 years who comprise about one-fifth of the total population
- Infants and young children also about one-fifth of the total population
- Old people who suffer more from chronic NCDs
- Contacts of people with infectious diseases, such as TB and Covid-19

- Agricultural and construction workers suffering hazards from machinery and dangerous chemicals.

Identifying risk factors also highlights the need to prevent and control risk exposures for NCDs, such as a high body-mass index for obesity, high systolic blood pressure for hypertension, high fasting plasma glucose for diabetes, dietary and nutritional risks, and unhealthy behaviours such as smoking tobacco, drinking alcohol, unsafe sex, and illicit drug use.

For equity it is also important to consider particular socio-economic and cultural groups such as:

- Marginal groups like poor families, women, disabled people, subsistence farmers, and migrants
- Ethnic groups or subgroups who are predisposed to ill health linked to their beliefs and customs
- People living remotely and far away from local health facilities
- People living in areas affected by large seasonal and climatic changes such as flooding
- Contacts of people with infectious diseases, such as TB and Covid-19
- Ethnic groups or subgroups who are systematically deprived of public services and predisposed to ill health, such as the 'tribal' peoples and the *Dalits* in India

14.8 Improving delivery of services

There is no standard way to measure and compare the provision of health care, but the four concepts of delivery, access, quality, and coverage are very important. Local health systems should aim to deliver to people the high-priority, high-quality, and effective health services and programmes that use guidelines based on international evidence and best practice. National health plans frequently include these in their national plans for the efficient and effective delivery of better services and programmes.

Achieving better equity is also critically important. For example, is it equitable for only 50% or a half of the district's population to live within 10 km of a health facility? Equity in local health planning requires analysis of the distribution and delivery of services and programmes in the whole district. Plans may have to include the establishment of new facilities or even expand the use of counselling, health, and welfare services.

Next steps are to estimate people's access to these services and programmes, and then to measure their quality and coverage. These four indicators measure how well the local management team is doing and whether the district is meeting its operational targets.

> IMPROVE DELIVERY, ACCESS, QUALITY, AND COVERAGE ALL
> HAVE HIGH PRIORITY

14.9 Improving access

Access is often stated as an objective in national health plans with priority for a high proportion of people to have access to a community health worker, health post, health centre, or hospital within 5 km or may be 10 km of their home (see Figure 14.2).

Access measures if households can obtain services and programmes that are also at acceptable levels of quality and coverage. Achieving high coverage is only possible if there is a good level of access. Coverage with interventions is

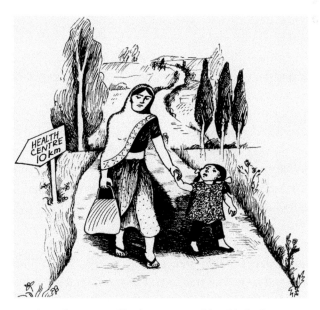

Figure 14.2 It takes 1 hour to walk 5 km to a rural health facility.

a measure of their effectiveness and an indication of whether they will lead to improved health outcomes and an improved health status.

A useful geographical method for estimating access is to calculate the percentage of people living within 5 km and 10 km of each facility (see Figure 15.3). When communications and transportation are poor, such as in rural and mountainous areas, distance is often used to reflect access. In urban areas and where transport is more available access is often defined in terms of time and costs. However, even if services are delivered locally it is important to also consider other costs like user fees and loss of earnings and wages. Social and cultural factors and seasonality changes may also be important when planning to improve access.

14.10 High-quality interventions

Achieving high-quality involves using health interventions that are organized to use evidence-based and recommended international standards and guidelines. Quality reflects how well these are being used and implemented. If quality is high then the service or programme will achieve higher levels of benefits, including for coverage (see Box 14.4).

Health interventions have to be organized and delivered to high evidence-based and recommended international standards and guidelines. Quality reflects how well these are being used and implemented. If quality is high then the service or programme will achieve higher levels of benefits. For instance, quality guidelines are available for communicable diseases such as for diarrhoea and TB. Achieving high quality involves using health interventions that are well organized and widely used and quality reflects how well these are being used and implemented. If quality is high then the service or programme will achieve higher levels of benefits, including coverage. However, high coverage can only be reached when inequalities are also tackled, which are discussed in Chapter 15 and Chapter 16.

Quality guidelines are widely available for many programmes, such as for family planning, reproductive health, child health, immunizations, communicable disease control for diarrhoea and TB, and NCDs including hypertension and diabetes. In addition, standards have been set for many of the inputs required for the health system itself, such as plans for health centre buildings, cold chains, and laboratory procedures.

The quality of services and programmes can be difficult to assess but they can be reviewed using a checklist of indicators and rapid qualitative methods,

Box 14.4 Monitoring for quality in TB control in Bangladesh

The World Health Organization (WHO, 2020) estimates that half of global TB cases are in eight high-burden countries: Bangladesh, China, India, Indonesia, Nigeria, Pakistan, the Philippines, and South Africa.

In Bangladesh in 1984, BRAC, a large non-governmental organization, began its TB control programme in one district. In 1994, with government agreement, it expanded its DOTS (directly observed treatment short course) programme across the country. This programme focuses on community education and household visits by Shebikas (community health workers) who refer people with a prolonged cough to the TB control services for sputum examination at local laboratories. They receive a small payment for detecting and caring for new cases.

Before starting on treatment new sputum-positive patients make a financial deposit which is returned if they successfully complete their treatment. Community stakeholder groups also help identify new TB patients and make sure that they take their own treatment. These groups include cured TB patients, religious leaders, school children, private practitioners, village doctors, and local pharmacists. Shebikas monitor patients to ensure they take their DOTS regularly and refer patients with complications to local health facilities.

In 2020, BRAC had 405 peripheral laboratories and 26 external quality assessment centres and its programme covered 297 sub-districts and 7 city corporations with a total population of over 92 million or 56% of the population of Bangladesh.

BRAC uses a range of **process indicators** to monitor the **quality** of its programme, including:

- Social support, home address, and mobile phone numbers
- Money collected and deposited from new patients
- Shebika incentives provided and payments made
- Sputum samples collected and dispatched
- New patients registered
- DOTS drugs made available and drug store maintenance
- Name of other different local providers of DOTS
- Quality of laboratory services
- Patient follow-up contacts and Shebika visits undertaken

The WHO's global and country monitoring helps to measure and track the global burden of TB. And its guidelines support countries conducting surveys to estimate indicators of health **outcome and impact,** such as TB incidence, morbidity, mortality, case-fatality ratio, treatment coverage, rifampicin and multidrug resistance, and latent TB infection in children under five years old.

Source data from http://www.brac.net/program/health-nutrition-and-population/tuberculosis-and-malaria-control/

such as exit interviews for patient satisfaction and focus groups for perceptions on how well services are organized (see Chapter 7).

14.11 Achieving high coverage

Coverage is an estimate of the proportion of all people in need of an intervention who actually receive it. This requires reliable data on the actual number of people who received the interventions (numerator) expressed as a percentage of the total number of people at risk in the target population (denominator). Interventions will be more effective if they are delivered with high quality and according to acceptable guidelines.

Achieving high levels of coverage is the single most important management objective. Other examples of important coverage indicators include the percentage of:

- People using masks as a preventive measure for Covid-19
- Births conducted by a skilled health worker
- 1–4-year-old children weighed regularly at child health clinics
- Diarrhoea patients receiving adequate oral rehydration therapy
- Pulmonary TB patients regularly receiving recommended treatment
- Married couples currently using a modern method of family planning
- Households with a safe water supply and latrines

Local coverage rates can be compared with the national rates and with other districts. However, national rates are usually an average for the whole country that can 'hide' wide variations between different districts. However, good local data from the routine information system, together with good judgement, are usually sufficient for most planning, management, monitoring, and evaluation purposes.

Special national surveys will be more accurate and may be required to assess a national programme. See Box 14.5 for an evaluation of a national immunization programme. To improve coverage requires that the main services and programmes are delivered, made accessible, and are of high quality. By estimating programme coverage the local team is also monitoring their own management. Coverage is a measure of how well the operational targets are being met and what targets need to be achieved the following year.

However, if coverage is thought to be reasonable and it can be maintained at the same level, the district health team might decide to give higher priority to improving another service or programme.

Box 14.5 Importance of achieving high coverage for child immunization

---

For child immunization the target population includes all live born infants under a year old. For example, in a population of say 200,000 people they are about 4% of the total or about 8,000 newborn infants in one year. If the district routine information system reported that 2,400 infants under one year had received three doses of diphtheria–pertussis–tetanus (DPT) vaccine during the year then the coverage is only 30%.

However, to reach the national average coverage of 45% the district health team has to improve its programme planning and management, especially if all districts are required to work towards the long-term national objective of 80% coverage.

If the district wants to reach the national objective of 80% coverage set by the national immunization programme it will need considerable improvements in the actual delivery, access, and quality. All these will need to improve. For instance, this might also include implementing more health education, use of mobile clinics, and expanding the immunization campaigns.

14.12 Local planning process

Health planning is a complicated and dynamic process that does not take place in a straightforward way. It is advisable, therefore, to select a few important issues and not attempt to be too comprehensive as this can risk new health plans not being implemented at all. The best approach is to tackle only two or three priority problems at a time. Guidance can often be sought from the national planning unit in the MOH or other credible professional groups.

If health teams have used all the available epidemiological information for planning they should have completed the following:

- Analysed the present situation, including for local health status
- Developed priorities for their next annual and medium-term plans
- Decided on which high-risk groups should receive priority
- Planned to improve delivery, access, quality, and coverage for the priority health programmes
- Decided on the objectives and main indicators needed to monitor and evaluate progress

When local health problems have been identified, priorities established, and the objectives and indicators chosen, the next step is to develop the framework for the medium-term plan. Detailed annual plans are the means to achieve the short-term objectives that are then included in the medium-term plans. When this process has been completed, the team should be in a good position to plan all the health services and programme activities that are needed to make the national health plans work in the district.

The following is a useful sequence for local planning and management. After deciding on the **priority problems**, next the team needs to decide on a **strategy**. For instance, if a priority is to reduce maternal mortality then the team might choose between improving access to the existing clinics, or establish new clinics, improving their quality, or reaching a higher coverage for supervised deliveries. This might also involve identifying more high-risk mothers, increasing the proportion of supervised deliveries at health centres, and training more midwives and traditional birth attendants.

Practical constraints may become clearer as the strategy is implemented and the team may then have to revise its original strategy. It can consult on the proposed strategy with MOH specialists and with community representatives, local government and councils, local NGOs, private practitioners, and other development sectors for their experience. Local leaders and politicians may be in a good position to give needed support.

Next the district team can **review all proposed activities** for their management implications regarding the required staffing, facilities, supplies, transport, and budgets. What are the implications for collaboration with other non-government health care providers?

Management then needs to establish and agree a **timetable** for activities and realistic start and completion dates. **Team members** can be assigned responsibility for carrying out the different activities and deciding on how to handle costs and budgets for both recurrent and capital costs.

Management also involves **communicating the strategy**. Do the staff understand the plan, main activities, and timetable? Is it clear which staff are incharge? Are maps, charts, and graphs understood?

Monitoring implementation and progress is essential. Is the plan working or are other modifications still required? Is the routine information system providing the relevant health data? Is epidemiological surveillance or a special survey required?

14.13 Summary of local health profile

The profile should contain a list of indicators for use in local health planning, management, and evaluation, including examples of the following:

District Population	Total	Age/sex groups	Births	Fertility
Health Status	Nutrition	Morbidity	Mortality	Rates
Health Resources	Facilities	Personnel	Finances	Training
Health Programmes	Pregnancy/delivery	Childcare		Environmental health

In support of UHC, the World Bank and the World Health Organization (WHO) have developed a framework to monitor progress, first by assessing the overall level and extent to which UHC is equitable, and secondly by whether national services and programmes offer service coverage and financial protection to all people within the population, including the poor and those living in remote areas.

The WHO recommends the use of the following 16 essential health services and programmes in 4 categories as indicators of the level and equity of coverage in countries:

1. **Reproductive, maternal, newborn, and child health:**
   - family planning
   - antenatal and delivery care
   - full child immunization
   - health-seeking behaviour for pneumonia

2. **Infectious diseases:**
   - TB treatment
   - HIV antiretroviral treatment
   - hepatitis treatment
   - use of insecticide-treated bed nets for malaria prevention
   - adequate sanitation

3. **Non-communicable diseases:**
   - prevention and treatment of raised blood pressure
   - prevention and treatment of raised blood glucose
   - cervical cancer screening
   - tobacco (non-)smoking

4. **Service capacity and access:**
   - basic hospital access
   - health worker density
   - access to essential medicines
   - health security: compliance with the International Health Regulations

15

Epidemiology for Monitoring
and Evaluation

15.1 What is monitoring and evaluation?

This chapter outlines how monitoring and evaluation can be used to analyse how well district health interventions, both services and programmes, are being implemented and their impact on health status. This is illustrated with practical and local examples on how this can be performed.

Monitoring involves the continuous measurement and observation of changes in the performance of the health services and programmes and their impact on the health status of populations to see whether they are being implemented according to national and local health plans. Management decisions are needed if monitoring reveals that there are problems with delivery, access, quality, or coverage. This can involve mid-course corrections to come back on track according to the original plan, and even changing strategies for services or programmes.

Evaluation attempts to determine as systematically and objectively as possible the relevance, effectiveness, and impact of activities in the light of their objectives. It determines whether the health plans have achieved the delivery as planned of interventions that can ultimately lead to improvements in health status. Evaluation is the starting point for a planning cycle that begins with an assessment of the achievements of the present national health policies and plans, followed by strengthening all activities that deliver health interventions as services and programmes by district and local health facilities. See Figure 1.6.

In the systems approach the priority is to monitor primary health care for the delivery of all the interventions and to evaluate whether they are achieving the agreed objectives for delivery, access, quality, and coverage.

INPUTS	PROCESSES	OUTPUTS	OUTCOMES	IMPACTS
Plan	Organize	Deliver	Achieve	Evaluate

This sequence involves a series of steps starting from national planning and working towards achieving local impact. There are four other important concepts that are used to evaluate what is being achieved.

Efficacy measures what an intervention or a package of interventions can achieve when carried out under near ideal circumstances, such as in randomized controlled trials. If preventive interventions are delivered at the highest levels by the services or programmes, including the highest levels of access, quality, and coverage, then health improvements should approach those achieved by efficacy.

Effectiveness measures what interventions actually achieve when implemented by health services or programmes. It measures what an intervention (e.g. measles vaccination) or a set of interventions (e.g. antenatal care) actually achieves when implemented by the routine health services or programmes.

Quality management aims to raise the level of effectiveness of a service or programme to be as near as possible to efficacy by performing according to the highest quality standards and guidelines. Quality management aims to reduce the gap between what can be achieved according to efficacy and what is actually achieved in practice. To achieve high quality requires well-trained staff performing to the agreed best standards and guidelines.

Efficiency is the relationship between programme inputs and outcomes. It is a measure of how efficiently the system converts inputs, such as staff, finances, and guidelines, in a cost-effective manner into the planned interventions and achieves the intended outcomes and impacts.

15.2 Monitoring equity and inequalities

Equity refers to fairness when planning the delivery of health services and programmes by ensuring that all citizens have good and equitable access to

Table 15.1 Infant mortality rate by household income quintile in South Africa (1993)

Household income quintile	Infant mortality rate per 1,000 live births
Poorest	86
Second	75
Third	60
Fourth	49
Richest	30
Rate ratio: poorest to richest quintile	2.9

Source data from L Gilson and D McIntyre, in T Evans et al (eds.): *Challenging inequities in health*. Oxford University Press (2001).

interventions. Experience shows, however, that this is hard to achieve as some people are more disadvantaged than others by such variables as their gender, age, socio-economic status, ethnicity, religion, and where they live. For instance, these variables can fundamentally affect indicators such as infant mortality rates.

An example of inequalities in South Africa is shown in Table 15.1 for infant mortality rates by household income quintiles. This shows that the mortality rate amongst the poorest people was nearly three times higher than for the richest people. When such equalities are identified corrective actions must be included in health policies. However, for any improvements to succeed requires that policies are well implemented for sufficient time periods, probably at least five years or more to see any substantial changes.

This example shows that children in the poorest quintile had a 2.9 times higher mortality than those in the wealthiest one. This ratio expresses relative inequality between the two extreme groups. A complementary way of presenting the gap is using absolute inequalities for the differences between two extreme groups. This shows that there were 56 more deaths for each 1,000 children per year in the poorest quintile compared to the wealthiest quintile. Such absolute gaps are often easier to interpret than relative gaps expressed as ratios.

Access to quality health services and programmes is critical if inequalities are to be reduced. Access is often measured by distance to the nearest health facilities and it is a fundamental indicator of inequalities. Regular monitoring helps to identify these differences.

Table 15.2 Percentage of Bangladeshi children aged 1–4 years who had any one of DPT, measles, or BCG vaccination by selected variables (% rounded)

Distance to health facility (miles)			Health worker visits in the last year		
< 1	2	3 or more	7 or more	1–6	None
32%	28%	21%	36%	27%	18%

Source data from ABBAS Bhuiya, Ismat Bhuiy, Mushtaque Chowdhury, Factors affecting acceptance of immunization among children in rural Bangladesh, Health Policy and Planning, Volume 10, Issue 3, September 1995, Pages 304–311, <https://doi.org/10.1093/heapol/10.3.304>

Table 15.2 shows inequities in immunization coverage in Bangladesh in the mid-1980s when the new Expanded Programme on Immunization (EPI) was first being implemented. Based on these findings the government and other agencies took corrective action to improve the immunization rates and this subsequently led to substantially reduced inequalities.

These figures clearly show the importance of inequalities in access as indicated by distance to the nearest health facility, influence of the child's gender (male 30%, female 25%), and wealth status of the family as indicated by possession of a household radio (Yes 37%, No 25%).

15.3 Monitoring delivery

Delivery is essential for present and future planning to obtain a fair and equitable distribution of health facilities, including for health centres, dispensaries, clinics, and community-based workers. Planning needs to keep pace with the health needs of the district population and also with local socio-economic developments. Are there any major gaps in the provision of health facilities and the services?

Consistently positive trends strongly suggest that a service is being delivered successfully. For instance, monitoring a positive trend in a frequency graph for antenatal care attendances or the supervision of health staff is good evidence of improved delivery (see Figure 15.1).

For example, in a district with 40 community health workers (at a low ratio of 1 per 5,000 people or approximately 1 per 1,000 households) the health team decided to visit CHWs for supervision and in-service monitoring once every 2 months, making 20 supervisions needed each month, and a total of 240 visits

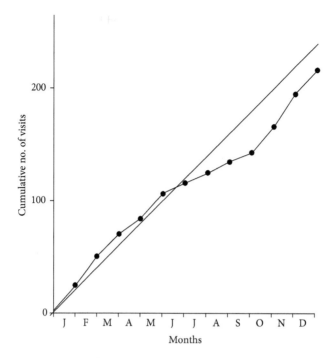

Figure 15.1 Supervision of community health workers

Reproduced with permission from Vaughan, J Patrick, Morrow, Richard H, and World Health Organization, Manual of epidemiology for district health management, World Health Organization; Geneva, Switzerland, Copyright © 1989

in one year. The monitoring graph in Figure 15.1 shows that this schedule started well but then slowed down and a special effort had then to be made to perform more supervision visits to catch up again on the planned schedule by the end of the year.

The graph in Figure 15.2 shows trend data for the number of mothers delivered at home per month by trained traditional birth attendants (TBAs) and by professional midwives in the district hospital and health centres.

Given a total of 8,000 deliveries per year in the district, the trained TBAs conducted and supervised 3,000 or 38% of all deliveries and midwives a further 1,900 or 24%, making a total of 62% of all births being attended to by a trained health worker. The graph also shows that deliveries by midwives rose more quickly over the year while the number deliveries by TBAs remained fairly constant. This information suggests that the public were more in favour of deliveries by the midwives.

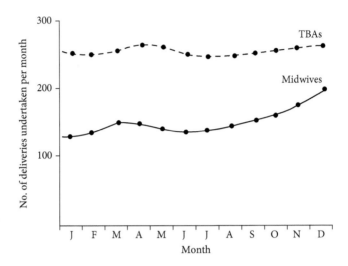

Figure 15.2 Monitoring home deliveries by trained traditional birth attendants (TBAs) and by professional midwives in local health centres and hospitals

Reproduced with permission from Vaughan, J Patrick, Morrow, Richard H, and World Health Organization, Manual of epidemiology for district health management, World Health Organization; Geneva, Switzerland, Copyright © 1989

15.4 Monitoring access

For greater equity and effective services it is critical to plan to deliver services to improve the population's access to local health facilities. Access is the most important output measure, particularly for all the interventions delivered at facilities such as health centres, clinics, and mobile clinics. In hilly and mountainous areas with a low population density and poor transportation access is often measured by distance, time, and costs while in urban areas time and costs are used more often.

A useful geographical method for estimating access is to calculate the percentage of people living within 5 km and 10 km of each facility. Figure 15.3 below shows that 75% or three-quarters of the district population live within 10 km and that only 50% or a half live within 5 km of their nearest health facility. Is it equitable and acceptable to have only a half of the district population having access to a health facility for family planning within 5 km of their home?

Other examples include access to safe water in or near houses and to sanitation. Both are important for the control of diarrhoeal diseases. Similarly, antenatal coverage will only be high if women have good local access to modern antenatal clinics at local health facilities or at mobile community clinics.

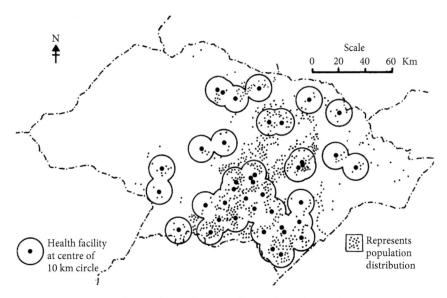

Figure 15.3 Map with population living within 10 km of a rural health facility.
Reproduced with permission from Vaughan, J Patrick, Morrow, Richard H, and World Health Organization, Manual of epidemiology for district health management, World Health Organization; Geneva, Switzerland, Copyright © 1989

15.5 Monitoring quality

High-quality health interventions are those that are judged to be evidence based and that use internationally agreed guidelines to deliver a high standard of health services and programmes. Evaluating quality means assessing whether these guidelines are being carefully followed and implemented. How well have the staff been trained to use them? How satisfied are patients and the public with the standard of care offered by these services?

Quality is usually assessed by direct observation and using a checklist of recommended procedures. See Chapter 7 for qualitative methods that can be used, such as direct observation, patient exit interviews, key informant interviews, and focus group discussions. These can provide useful qualitative insights and assessments. However, observations using these methods can also be subjective and care is needed to minimize bias by both the patients and observers. It is best if the quality assessment can be given as an estimated percentage value, such as 10%, 30%, 50%, 70%, or 90%, so this value can be used in calculating the overall community effectiveness and performance of a service or programme. For example, see Box 14.4 for monitoring immunization and the effect of low quality.

15.6 Monitoring coverage

Estimating district population coverage is the most critical indicator for the equitable distribution of interventions. Health teams must consider all people who could benefit from the intervention(s) and not only those people who attended the service(s). Coverage of the population is defined as the percentage or proportion of the target population (denominator) in the whole district population who are in need of a procedure or intervention compared to those who have actually received it (numerator).

For example, coverage of interventions can be measured for all individuals (e.g. immunizations for infants) or for a package of interventions (e.g. antenatal care for pregnant mothers). The target populations must be defined for each single health-related intervention and for the whole package of different interventions. The target population for immunization is all live-born infants under one year old and for antenatal care it includes all pregnant women. For example, in a district population of 200,000 people and an estimated 8,000 infants under one year old for immunization, the target group (denominator population), the coverage is the percentage of the 8,000 children who are fully immunized (numerator) before their first birthday during the past year as shown in Box 14.4.

For some interventions additional information may be needed. For example, to estimate the annual coverage for anti-tuberculosis (TB) treatment, the number of TB cases receiving or having completed treatment in the last 12 months (numerator) should be known from the routine information system. However, the target population (denominator) may have to be an estimate based on the expected total number of all new cases of pulmonary TB expected in the same population during the year. This depends on using a good estimate of the incidence for new TB cases in the local population.

15.7 Evaluating impact of interventions

High quality of care depends on using evidence-based guidelines, well trained and reliable health staff, and good management support for the health systems. These are illustrated by the evaluation of WHO IMCI (Integrated Management of Child Illnesses) guidelines that was conducted in Tanzania in 2000. The question was how effective were the interventions when they were delivered by routine health services and programmes (see Box 15.1).

Box 15.1 Evaluating impact of IMCI Care in Tanzania

Integrated Management of Child Illnesses (IMCI) was a new WHO-proposed package of interventions and evidence was needed on its effectiveness for quality and outcomes. Health impact as measured by infant and child mortality requires good epidemiological methods and a long period of implementation before impact can be evaluated whereas outcomes can be measured more quickly.

A health facility survey was carried out in Tanzania in 2000 to assess quality of care and health systems support for case management. The evaluation research team visited a representative sample of 75 first-level government health facilities in two districts where health workers had been trained in IMCI patient management and another two districts where health workers had not yet been trained in IMCI.

The team spent one day in each facility and observed the case management of total of 419 children based on the first 6 sick children aged 2 months to 5 years whose caretaker agreed to take part. They were interviewed again on exiting the facility and children were also examined again by an IMCI-trained 'gold standard; physician. Children were checked for three danger signs: cough, diarrhoea, and fever, and also weighed and checked against a growth chart.

Results showed that children in IMCI districts received better quality of care than children in the comparison districts. Their health problems were more thoroughly assessed and they were more likely to be correctly diagnosed and treated based on the 'gold-standard' re-examination. IMCI treatment of sick children included: (i) whether oral antibiotics and anti-malarial medicines were correctly prescribed, and (ii) whether children leaving the facility had been correctly prescribed antibiotics or not.

Supervisory visits in the six months before the survey were reported by almost all the health facilities although actual observation of case management was much more common in the IMCI districts. Health workers trained up to three years before the survey performed just as well as those trained more recently, and junior health staff trained in IMCI performed just as well as their more senior colleagues. Although case management for malaria was much improved in IMCI districts, the health impact was probably limited due to the high levels of chloroquine drug resistance in the districts.

The findings showed that children in the IMCI districts received more appropriate treatment and caretakers reported better knowledge about caring for their sick children, when to return again to the clinic, and how to correctly give oral medications. All differences were statistically significant (p < 0.05). However, there were few significant differences between the IMCI and comparison districts for support by the health systems.

Source: Impact of IMCI health worker training on routinely collected child health indicators in Northeast Brazil. Amaral J et al. Health Policy Plan, 2005, 20 Suppl 1, 42–48.

Reproduced from Amaral J, Leite AJ, Cunha AJ, Victora CG. Impact of IMCI health worker training on routinely collected child health indicators in Northeast Brazil. Health Policy Plan. 2005 Dec;20 Suppl 1:i42-i48. doi: 10.1093/heapol/czi058. with permission from Oxford University Press

15.8 Evaluating programme effectiveness

Programme effectiveness measures how well routine local health systems deliver high-priority interventions within health services and programmes. Evidence for the effectiveness of interventions is often based on community quasi-experimental trials that involve whole populations rather than trials based on individuals.

The actual effectiveness and performance of a service or programme is the product of *quality × coverage × efficacy* when implementation is carried out under routine conditions. This is illustrated in Box 15.2.

Box 15.2 Measuring the effectiveness of a district measles immunization programme

The quality of an immunization programme was assessed and the programme coverage was found to be high at 80% for measles vaccination among infants. The efficacy of measles vaccination is known to be 95% under best circumstances among non-immune infants. Few infants will have been infected with the measles virus before one year old.

To review programme quality direct observation was used which showed that the performance of the health staff was inadequate and that overall quality was assessed to be low due to poor quality control of the cold chain, incorrect vaccination procedures and only 50% of the doses being administered correctly. Quality was estimated, therefore, to be only 50%.

Programme effectiveness = quality x coverage x efficacy = 0.5 x 0.8 x 0.95 = 0.38 or 38%

This means that in fact only 38% of infants were protected and not the expected 95%. While population coverage appeared to be acceptable, the quality and management of the programme was much too low and urgently had to be corrected. Retraining of staff was needed if quality was to be raised back up to a satisfactory level.

This example shows that effectiveness depends on the following five factors:

- Efficacy of the intervention as determined by randomized controlled trials
- Delivery of interventions to the whole population in need
- Access to interventions by the whole target group in the population
- High-quality interventions are well implemented and organized
- High coverage is achieved in the target population

High-quality management is needed to achieve an equitable and fair distribution of services within the whole population in the district. This aims to raise the level of effectiveness of a service or programme to be as close as possible to efficacy by performing according to the highest quality standards and guidelines. The aim is to reduce the gap between what can be achieved according to efficacy and what is actually being achieved in practice. Achieving high coverage for the whole district population requires that interventions are delivered, accessible, and are of high quality. This needs well-trained staff performing to evidence-based standards and guidelines.

Effectiveness also depends on the efficiency of the programme and how well its inputs are converted into outputs, such as use of vaccines, staff, finances, and guidelines. To achieve the required outcomes the interventions must then be successfully organized and delivered with high levels of access.

15.9 Monitoring equity and health inequalities

It is important that health data is analysed and monitored for inequalities and that, as discussed in Chapter 14, health plans take a long-term view towards achieving improvements in health status. For example, to achieve reductions in inequalities among different groups in the population can take many years and high levels of coverage are essential. It is clearly important in health planning therefore to analyse disaggregated health data in order to make equitable and fair decisions. It is important to monitor coverage with an equity lens and to know that inequalities can be reduced with the right health policies and over time.

Figure 15.4 shows how Cambodia made progress in providing antenatal care to women from poorer families. Each circle shows coverage by wealth

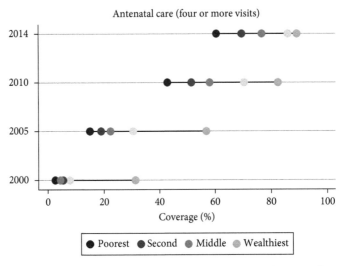

Figure 15.4 Cambodia antenatal care for four or more visits by quintile groups 2000–2014

Source: Exemplars in Global health: Under-5 Mortality: Cambodia Study, Hirschhorn, LR. et al. 2020

quintiles for the national population, starting from the poorest 20% (dark circle) households to the richest 20% (light circle) households. In the year 2000 antenatal coverage for the lowest four groups for visits was close to zero but over 14 years antenatal coverage increased to over 60% for the poorest group. It increased in all five wealth groups. The order of the groups did not change although the gap between them did decrease. However, even with this improvement the coverage gap between the poorest and wealthiest quintiles was still about 30% points. This is a typical pattern often seen for improvements in inequalities.

Cambodia also achieved remarkable falls in both neonatal and under-five year mortality (U5M) despite challenges in both regional access and coverage for its child health services and programmes. As well as improving their access and coverage success was also due to a strong commitment to tackling social determinants of health, such as economic growth, female empowerment, stunting, poverty reduction, and WASH. These were also all key factors influencing mortality. In addition, improving overall health status required strong national leadership and health systems strengthening, together with partner financial resources to support these interventions. However, despite these efforts challenges still remained for equity in access and coverage to neonatal health services and with the necessary strengthening of human health resources.

Such equity analysis requires large-scale surveys carried out every five years or so. These are best carried out by specialist research centres and not by districts themselves. However, simpler analyses can be undertaken by district teams, such as differences in access for boys and girls, access for rural and urban populations, and for those with no schooling compared to those completing primary level,

15.10 Ethics and equity in health planning

The health system is responsible for all people living in the districts who could benefit from interventions, and it is not equitable or fair or just to deliver good services only to those people who live near facilities or the wealthy ones who can afford to pay fees and for transport. Although improving delivery, access, and quality are necessary to achieve high levels of population coverage, low access and poor-quality services can be unethical and lead to inequity due to lower coverage and inefficient services which can result in higher costs per unit of service.

Achieving equity by health services and programmes has to be a priority although this can raise difficult choices. Achieving fair delivery, high access, good quality and acceptable coverage for all people in a district has to be aimed for but clearly can be difficult to achieve. For instance, it is more difficult to deliver services in remote areas and for poor and deprived people. However, underserved populations often have greater health needs than those who already have good access. It is also easier to favour the demands of wealthier people living near health facilities. New investments can be justified on the basis of achieving better equity.

Equity also involves quality management that aims to be more efficient by reducing costs. The costs of poor management can be obvious, such as poorly maintained buildings, broken equipment, long waiting times for patients, and insufficient stocks of essential drugs. There are also administrative costs to training staff, maintaining transport, and health educating the community. However, other costs are less apparent or transparent, such as time wasted by patients, lack of public trust, unused medications, and poor-quality services. These can lead to clinical complications and even deaths.

The World Bank and the World Health Organization (WHO) have developed a framework to track the progress of UHC by monitoring the overall level and the extent to which UHC is equitable as well as whether it offers service coverage and financial protection to all people in the population, including the poor and disadvantaged. The WHO has recommended 16 essential health services in 4 categories as indicators of the level and equitable coverage in countries (see Section 14.12).

16

Using Ethical Principles

16.1 Why are ethics important?

Ethics helps health planners to be fair and just when making choices on priorities in health planning by using these principles, values, and guidelines to help decide between possible 'right' and 'wrong' planning decisions that can benefit both individuals and communities. These principles have international agreement. In addition, these are linked to global human rights, such as the United Nations Declaration on Human Rights and the UN Rights of the Child which have been accepted and ratified by most countries. An example of restricting individual freedoms in epidemics is given in Box 16.1.

All health workers should make best use of ethical principles in decision-making, whether employed in government, non-government, or private services. These ethical principles have wide international agreement. Countries also have their own separate national laws and regulations to protect the rights of their citizens. With international debate these ethical principles, guidelines, and values can change over time as new scientific knowledge evolves and new technologies become available.

The CIOMS—Council for International Organisations of Medical Sciences—is a non-governmental, non-profit organization established jointly by the World Health Organization (WHO) and the United Nations Educational, Scientific and Cultural Organization (UNESCO) in 1949. The mission of the CIOMS is to advance public health through guidance on health research and policy, including on ethics, medical product development, and safety (see Annex Five). It represents the biomedical and scientific communities through its member organizations, which include many of the biomedical disciplines, national academies of sciences, and medical research councils.

Box 16.1 Individual freedom of movement and controlling epidemics

---

Ethics considers the benefits of restricting travel in an epidemic when the benefits are sufficiently great to outweigh infringements on the rights of individuals. However, the benefits should be seen to be strong to outweigh any drastic restrictions and should, if possible, apply to everyone in the area.

For example, in controlling Ebola or Covid-19 epidemics the right to travel might be restricted or stopped altogether by governments imposing lockdowns. People's movements may also be restricted by quarantine measures imposed on ill people, any suspected cases, contacts, or travellers.

Most people agree that this is ethically justified to control epidemics and to protect other people from becoming infected. The benefits of stopping the epidemic are seen to outweigh the loss of individual freedoms. However, restricting the rights of people with TB or HIV/AIDS to travel is not usually seen as acceptable.

Public messages must be clear and adhered to by everyone unless people are exempt. Mixed and unclear messaging to the public must be avoided.

16.2 Ethical principles

With limited resources there can be tensions between the needs of individuals, such as for individual freedoms, and wanting a better local hospital or individual household water supplies, or competing priorities by public health programmes like tuberculosis (TB) control and child immunization.

The following four ethical principles are recognized internationally and they apply equally in both public and private health services and for both individuals and whole communities. These principles are particularly important when used in public health programmes:

- Autonomy: Respecting individual's rights and allowing them to make informed choices
- Justice: Achieving a fair and equitable distribution of benefits and risks in the population

- Beneficence: Producing benefits that far outweigh risks
- Non-maleficence: Avoiding any undue harm or injury

If one principle has to take precedence and override another it is important to be clear why and which one has priority. Clarity also helps to reduce public controversy and to maintain public trust in government policies.

Autonomy—This is the right of individuals to be in charge of decisions regarding their own health. It means giving priority to informed consent, privacy, confidentiality, and the right to access health information. Autonomy can present difficulties and be reduced by illnesses like dementia, head injuries, or schizophrenia, and autonomy of children, women, elderly, and disabled may also be compromised or reduced. Children only gain full legal autonomy on reaching adulthood.

Justice—This concerns the fair and equitable distribution of benefits and risks and means that all people should be given equal access to acute services, treatment facilities, and preventive health programmes. Justice and equity are basic principles in health, including achieving spatial or geographical justice. Justice is also concerned with the fair allocation of local health care resources and people's inability to pay fees for clinic and hospital services. Justice aims to avoid discrimination, particularly that due to poverty, gender, and disabilities.

Beneficence—Benefits must outweigh risks in all curative services and all public health programmes. These should achieve much more good than harm. Harm varies from the severe, such as quarantine and surgery, to minimal such as giving a vaccine or completing a questionnaire. In general, people and communities will accept harm if they believe that it leads to more good than more harm. For example, communities may believe that the benefits of insecticide spraying are marginal compared to the inconvenience caused to them and people may be unlikely to test for human immunodeficiency virus/acquired immunodeficiency syndrome (HIV/AIDS) when no local treatment services are available. A clear positive balance for benefits over harm is important in all public health programmes.

Non-maleficence—This means that health staff and services should practice to the highest professional standards in order to avoid doing any undue harm to individuals or communities. For instance, health data need to be collected for the benefit of all individuals as well as for the whole community. This principle is often linked to beneficence.

ETHICS HELPS PLANNING MAKE JUST AND FAIR CHOICES

16.3 Using ethical principles

Although ethical principles for individuals are widely agreed there is less agreement on their use for public health programmes and in community interventions. See Annex Five for research studies.

Confidentiality

Health workers are responsible for ensuring confidentiality at all times for health records and should know the national ethical and legal rules for accessing private health data. No individuals should be identified in public reports although some anonymous data, such as the prevalence of raised blood pressure or incidence of new HIV/AIDS cases, can be published. Publishing data on poor households and high-risk groups can also be problematic since it is important to avoid causing public prejudice, alarm, and stigmatization. Ownership and confidentiality of data and records vary between countries.

Informed consent

People are free to accept or refuse clinical or preventive procedures, such as an operation or a vaccination, and they must be informed about any risks before giving consent. They are also free not to accept to participate in a treatment, survey, or intervention trial (see Box 16.2).

Dignity and privacy

Health staff should treat patients with full respect, dignity, and courtesy. Hospitals and clinics should have good waiting areas and private clinic rooms to ensure confidential interviews and clinical examinations. Women may need to be chaperoned. And it is totally unacceptable for staff to ask for gifts, money, or favours in exchange for services.

Patient records may be kept confidential in hospitals and clinics, while in many countries they are kept by patients at home, such as clinic or vaccination cards for mothers and children.

Box 16.2 Guidelines on information required for informed consent

Informed consent ensures that people and patients know what they can expect if they agree to participate in clinical treatment, a public health procedure, or a research study. They should also know that they are free to refuse and withdraw at any time. All procedures for patients and participants must be fully explained. They can also involve a relative or friend before agreeing.

Sometimes individuals and women may not be free to give consent. If permission is agreed by community leaders, individuals are still free to refuse to participate. There may be serious issues if people are not free to consent.

Research studies and special procedures are covered by ethical procedures (see Annex Five).

Informed consent and the following information must be clearly and fully explained:

- What is the procedure, research, or study about?
- Who is doing the study and why is it being done?
- What procedures will be used, for example, questionnaires, blood samples, tissue biopsies?
- Number of attendances needed, where, and who performs interviews and examinations?
- Any risks and discomfort involved, including pain and possible side effects
- Benefits to participating, for example, health care, drugs or treatments, education, rewards
- Participants can refuse and are free to withdraw at any time with no risk or penalties
- For laboratory specimens explain what will be done with them and any tissue remains
- Who owns the resulting information and intellectual property rights?
- Contact names for information and quality control to answer any questions

Individual and community levels

Autonomy refers to the right of individuals to make decisions that affect their own life and health. A full explanation of what will be entailed in a given event or intervention and answering patient questions encourage public trust. Health workers also need to respect people as equal partners in both curative care and in public health programmes.

Respect for autonomy

Ethics helps people and health workers make good decisions, although for children decisions are often taken by parents or carers. Autonomy may also be impaired for people with poor mental health or with severe psychiatric illness, coma, illicit drug use, and alcohol abuse. Autonomy may also be impaired for marginalized and poor communities, women, minority ethnic groups, nomads, and street children. However, if at all possible they should be included in any decisions that affect them.

Restricting individual freedom

The global Covid-19 pandemic has led many countries to restrict individual freedoms such as imposing lockdown, curfews, isolation, and quarantines. To encourage public trust such restrictions should be seen to be fair and be widely explained in the mass media, social networks, radio, and television. Where possible restrictions should be explained in writing, lifted as soon as possible, apply equally to everyone in designated areas and all those with the same conditions.

Vulnerability

People's vulnerability can be affected by their social status and where and how they live. Are the disadvantaged and vulnerable all benefiting equally from local services? Is equity included in the analysis of health information? For example, poor people living in rural areas often have higher disease burdens and also suffer by having less access to services than their wealthier counterparts living in urban areas. Illiteracy and poverty can affect people's ability to understand health information and advice. People's autonomy can also be reduced by cultural norms and beliefs, as well as by religious practices, repressive laws, and by food insecurity.

> **ALL PEOPLE ARE ENTITLED TO INFORMED CONSENT**

16.4 Ethics and equity in health planning

Health equity—or equity in health—is defined as the absence of unfair and avoidable or remediable differences in health status among population groups defined socially, economically, demographically, or geographically. Barriers that limit access of some population groups to quality health services and public health programmes must be removed in order to achieve health equity.

Equity in health is concerned with achieving fairness and impartiality in health outcomes. Equity involves equal access to high-quality health services and public health programmes, regardless of people's location and their socio-economic, ethnic, and cultural status.

Health inequalities measure the differences in health outcomes, for example, between health indicators for different socio-economic groups, such as rich and poor people or men and women or those living close to and far from health facilities. Planning should aim to be fair and just when trying to reduce health inequalities. This means being fair to all people and not just the wealthier people and those living near the health services! And if possible, all people should be given equal and the same priority.

However, planning also involves choosing between priority interventions to reduce inequalities for different health problems and even giving higher priority to some at risk population groups. National priorities are often selected by national planning units in the Ministry of Health based on scientific evidence and their costs and feasibility.

There is good agreement on the ethical principles and guidelines for personal health services but these ethical principles apply equally to government, non-government, and private health care providers. There may be less clarity on their application in non-personal and public health programmes. But all services and programmes need to respect human rights and dignity, enhance people's autonomy, and support the poorest and most vulnerable. For example, the disadvantaged can include the poor, women, marginal ethnic groups, people living in remote areas, people with disabilities, and those affected by marked seasonal changes.

> **IN PLANNING EVERY EFORT MUST BE MADE TO BE FAIR AND JUST**

Wherever possible, people should also be involved in, or at least represented, in health planning decisions and it is not acceptable to favour some individuals, families, and communities more than others. Promoting equity requires good-quality local health data and information on disadvantaged groups. It is also important to be aware that using data that are selective and unrepresentative of the total population is by itself unethical. There are also important ethical issues when analysing and using poor-quality health data to make planning decisions. Using fake or poor-quality data is totally unethical.
Promoting greater equity to reduce inequalities involves:

- The fair delivery and distribution of health services, programmes, and staff across the district
- Ensuring access to all services for everyone within a reasonable distance and at affordable costs
- Enabling high-quality services and programmes to be performed to acceptable quality guidelines
- Achieving high levels of population coverage for all priority interventions
- Promoting health financing that is fairly distributed between curative and preventive services, between urban and rural populations, and between administration and systems support

Promoting equity definitely requires that population health information is disaggregated by wealth, gender, ethnicity, place of residence, and any other relevant characteristics for sub-groups.

> **PROMOTING EQUITY REQUIRES REPRESENTATIVE HEALTH INFORMATION**

16.5 Ethics for health research

Internationally approved guidelines exist for the conduct and organization of epidemiological health studies and research and intervention studies. These include the best ethical practices and the rights of the participants involved. More information is available from Internet websites and in Annex Five.

Most countries have procedures and committees for the ethical review of all health research proposals. Research studies involving local populations will usually need Research Ethics Committee (REC) clearance and formal and written approval. While routine health procedures may not require review, research studies involving patients or general population surveys usually do require ethical review and approval by a nationally recognized REC before research can start. This committee is often organized by the national ministry of health, medical research council or an established university. More details on ethical review are available in Annex Five and from Internet websites.

Acceptable incentives for participation in research for research participants can include a small financial support for travel, food and refreshment, and perhaps money to replace income lost due to participating in an investigation. These are only to compensate for small costs incurred. Some studies also offer small incentives, such as a toy or gadget, to encourage people to participate or remain in a study but these should be small enough that people feel free to refuse to participate. Large benefits compared to the participants' normal incomes are unethical. They are undue incentives which can appear to be bribe.

17

ABC of Common Definitions and Terms

A

Access. The proportion of a defined population that has a particular health facility within reasonable reach; this is often measured by using distance (e.g. 5 km or 10 km), time (e.g. within 2 hours walk), or costs (e.g. free or with user charges). Economic, social, and cultural factors must also be taken into account.

Accuracy. The degree to which a measured value represents the true value of the variable being measured. For diagnostic tests, the ability of the test to correctly classify the presence or absence of the target disorder. See Repeatability and Validity.

Agent. A factor whose presence or deficiency is essential for the occurrence of a disease, for example microorganisms, protozoa, chemical substances, vitamins, or essential amino acids.

Age-sex pyramid. See Population pyramid.

Age-specific rate. A rate for a specified age group, based on using the numerator and denominator for the same age group. The 1–4 child mortality rate, for instance, is calculated using the number of deaths among 1–4 year olds in a specified population and area during one year as a numerator, multiplied by 1,000 and divided by the average total population aged 1–4 years in the same area during the same year (denominator).

Age standardization. A procedure for adjusting rates (e.g. death rates), designed to minimize the effects of differences in the age composition of two or more populations. See Annex One.

Airborne infection. A disease caused by an infectious agent that can be transmitted by particles or droplets suspended in the air, for example measles pertussis and Covid-19.

Anthropometry. Technique for measuring size, weight, height, and body proportions in humans.

Antibody. Protein molecule formed in response to exposure to a 'foreign' or extraneous substance, such as microorganisms; the presence or concentration of antibodies is usually noted and measured in the blood or serum.

Antigen. A substance (protein, polysaccharide, glycolipid, or tissue graft) that can induce a specific antibody response, such as with infectious organisms and vaccines. See Immunization.

Arbovirus. A group of animal viruses transmitted to humans by blood-feeding arthropod vectors, for example mosquitoes, ticks, sandflies, and midges. The term is an abbreviation of 'arthropod-borne virus'.

Asset index. A frequently used measure of the socioeconomic position of a household, derived from the presence of assets (e.g. radio, television, smartphones) and building characteristics (e.g. materials used in the floor, walls, and roof; presence of piped water and electricity). Using a statistical method known as principal component analyses, a single index measure is derived from these characteristics, and all households in a sample are ranked into wealth quintiles, from the poorest 20% to the wealthiest 20%. See Percentiles.

Association. Statistical dependence between two or more variables; these are said to be associated if they occur together more frequently than would be expected by chance. Statistical tests enable the degree and level of significance of the association to be calculated.

Attack rate. This rate usually refers to the incidence of new cases during an epidemic. The secondary attack rate is based on the number of new cases among contacts of a primary case that occur within the accepted incubation period of the disease. The denominator is the total number of exposed contacts during the same period of time. An attack rate above 1.0 indicates that the number of cases is increasing in the population. See Secondary attack rate and Reproductive rate.

Attributable risk. The rate or proportion of a disease or other outcome in exposed individuals that can be attributed to the particular exposure; it is calculated by subtracting the rate of the outcome (usually incidence or mortality) among the unexposed from the outcome rate among those exposed.

Autonomy. The ethical principle of respect for human dignity and the right for individuals to decide for themselves. This is essential for informed choice and informed consent.

Average. See Mean, arithmetic

Axis. One dimension in a graph. A two-dimensional graph has two axes, x on the horizontal and y on the vertical.

B

Behavioural risk factor. A characteristic or behaviour associated with an increased risk of specified outcomes, although this may not be a causal association.

Bias. Any effect during the collection or interpretation of information that leads to a systematic error in one direction, for example errors resulting from weighing scales under-recording a child's true weight, or observer bias in the interpretation of replies to questions in a questionnaire. Bias represents a systematic deviation of results or inferences from truth. See Error.

Birth rate. A summary crude rate based on the number of live births in a known population over a given period of time.

$$\text{Birth rate} = \frac{\text{Number of live births in area during one year}}{\text{Average total population in area during the same year}} \times 1{,}000$$

Birth weight. Infant's weight recorded at the time of birth. Low birth weight babies weigh less than 2500 grams and the percentage of such babies is commonly used as a measure of maternal undernutrition, or more broadly of population health.

Blind study. A single blind study is one in which either observers or subjects do not know which groups the subjects are assigned to, such as in a trial, or who are the cases or controls in an observational or non-intervention study. A double blind study means both subjects and observers are unaware which groups the subjects belong to. The intent of keeping subjects and/ or investigators blinded (i.e. unaware of knowledge that might introduce a bias) is to reduce the likelihood of such bias.

C

Carrier. A person or animal that harbours a specific infectious agent in the absence of clinical disease and that constitutes a potential source for further transmission of the infection.

Case. A person identified as having a particular characteristic, for example a disease, behaviour, or condition. The epidemiological definition of a case is not necessarily the same as the clinical definition. Cases may be divided into possible, probable, and definite, depending on how well-specific criteria are satisfied.

Case-control study. An analytical epidemiological study that compares cases of a particular condition with suitable control subjects who do not have the condition, looking at the frequency of associated factors (often 'risk factors') in the two groups. Often used to test hypotheses about aetiology, for example the link between lung cancer and cigarette smoking. These studies do not reveal causation.

Case-fatality rate. The percentage of persons dying from a given condition during a given time period, expressed as a proportion of all those contracting the condition during that period. This rate is most commonly used for communicable diseases. Not to be confused with the mortality rate.

Case-fatality rate
$$= \frac{\text{Number of deaths from a disease in a given period}}{\text{Number of cases of disease diagnosed in the same period of time}} \times 100$$

Case-finding. A standard procedure to locate and treat people who have or who have been in close contact with a known case, usually an infectious disease. Also, seeking persons who have been exposed to risk of other potentially harmful factors,

Catchment area. The geographical area from which the people attending a particular health facility come.

Census. The enumeration of an entire population, usually with details on residence, age, sex, occupation, ethnic group, marital status, birth history, and relationship to head of household. A *de facto* census only counts the people who are actually present during the enumeration; a *de jure* census records all people according to their normal place of residence at the time of enumeration.

Chemoprophylaxis. The administration of drugs to prevent an infection from occurring or to prevent the infection from progressing into disease.

Child mortality rate. Number of annual deaths in children aged less than 5 years old (numerator) expressed as a rate per 1,000 live births in that year; often both numerator and denominator are averaged over the previous 5 years.

Class. A group of observations made on a variable, considered together for the convenience of analysis, for example, haemoglobin values may be classed by intervals of one g/100 ml.

Classification of diseases. Arrangement of diseases into agreed and standard groups, for example in the International Classification of Diseases published by the World Health Organization.

Clustering. The grouping of a series of cases in relation to time or spatial area, or both. During an outbreak or epidemic, the space-time clustering of cases commonly suggests a point-source outbreak due to an infectious agent or toxic chemical.

Cluster sampling. A sampling method in which each unit selected is composed of a group of persons, for example villages and households, rather than an individual.

Cohort. A well-defined group of people who have had a common experience or exposure and are then followed up for the incidence of new diseases or events (cohort or prospective study). A group of people born during a particular period or year is called a birth cohort.

Communicable period. The time during which an infectious agent may be transferred from an infected person or animal to another susceptible person or animal or vice versa.

Confounding. The distortion of a measure of the effect of an exposure on an outcome due to the association of the exposure with other factors that influence the occurrence of the same outcome. Confounding occurs when all or part of the apparent association between the exposure and outcome is in fact accounted for by other variables that affect the outcome and are not themselves affected by exposure. For example, prevalence of overweight may be higher among children living in homes with a microwave oven than in the rest of the child population, but this may be due to higher socio-economic position of their families, and not because eating microwaved food leads to overweight. See confounding bias.

Contact. Exposure to a source of an infection. Transmission due to direct contact may occur when skin or mucous membranes touch, as in body contact, such as kissing and sexual intercourse; indirect contact may occur through transmission by aerosols or respiratory droplets, or by touching contaminated objects.

Contagious. Transmitted by contact or close proximity.

Control group. Subjects with whom comparison is made in a case-control study, a randomized controlled trial, or other epidemiological study. In a case-control or cross-sectional study, controls are people who do not present the disease or outcome being studied. In a randomized controlled trial, controls are the individuals who do not receive the intervention being tested. Instead they may receive a placebo or no treatment. See case-control studies; cross-sectional surveys; randomized controlled trial.

Control programmes. Disease control programmes aim to lower the incidence of new cases or reduce the proportion of severe cases through treatment or other interventions, to an acceptably low level so that the disease is no longer considered a major public health hazard.

Correlation. The degree to which variables change together. A correlation coefficient is a measure of association that indicates the degree to which two or more sets of observations fit a linear or straight-line relationship. Correlation may be positive, when both variables increase together, or negative, when one increases as the other decreases.

Cost. The value of resources engaged in providing a service. Average cost per unit refers to the total costs divided by the total number of units provided.

Coverage. A measure of the ratio of people or households who have actually received a particular service compared to all those who need it, usually expressed as a percentage, for example, of households with a reasonably safe water supply, percentage of infants immunized with three doses of DPT vaccine, or percentage of deliveries attended by a skilled birth atendant.

$$\text{Coverage with skilled birth attendance} = \frac{\text{Number of deliveries attended by a skilled birth attendant}}{\text{Expected number of deliveries in same population during same period}} \times 100$$

Cross-sectional survey. A survey or study that examines people in a defined population at one point in time. Cross-sectional surveys usually supply prevalence data but repeated surveys can be used to give an estimate of incidence. Cross-sectional surveys may also be used to study how the prevalence of a health outcome such as high blood pressure varies according to different risk factors or physical activity.

Cumulative incidence. The number or proportion of a group of people who experience the onset of a health-related event during a specified time period, such as new cases of Covid-19 in a defined population over one year. This interval is generally the same for all members of the group, but as in lifetime incidence it may vary from person to person without reference to the age at which the event occurs; for example, cumulative mortality due to breast cancer in a birth cohort of 1,000 women. Also known as 'incidence proportion'. See Incidence.

D

Data processing. Conversion of raw data into a form suitable for analysis with computers and statistical programmes.

Death rate. The proportion of a population who die from any cause during a specified period of time. The rate can be made specific for a particular cause or group of causes of death. The rate can also be calculated separately for each sex and any age group, thus providing disease-, sex- and age-specific rates.

Crude death rate

$$= \frac{\text{Number of all deaths during one year}}{\text{Average total population during same year (or mid-year population)}} \times 1,000$$

Demand for health care. Willingness and/or ability to seek and use services. Sometimes further divided into expressed demand or actual use, and potential demand or need. Financial, geographic, or cultural barriers may limit the ability to use services.

Demography. The study of populations, with reference to such factors as size, age structure, density, fertility, mortality, migration, growth, ethnic, and socio-economic characteristics.

Demographic transition. The transition in a population from high to low fertility and mortality rates. It is accompanied by a change in the age composition of the population as birth rates and death rates decline. These trends result in a decrease in the proportion of children and young adults and an increase in the proportion of older persons in the population.

Denominator. The lower portion of a fraction. In the calculation of a rate, this represents the total population at risk.

Disability-Adjusted Life Years (DALYs). A summary measure of the burden of disease in a defined population. It may be used to estimate the effectiveness of interventions. DALYs are based on adjusting life expectancy by including disease incidence and discounting periods of life lived with disability. 'Disability weights' are multiplied by the period due to disability or chronological age to reflect the burden of the disability.

Disease, subclinical. The condition in which a disease is only detectable by special tests and there are no apparent clinical symptoms and signs.

E

Effectiveness. A measure of how well specific interventions, procedures, regimens, or services used in services and ordinary programmes actually achieve what they are supposed to do. Effective relates to how well programmes or interventions work in real life. See efficacy.

Efficacy. The extent to which a specific intervention, procedure, regimen, or service produces a beneficial result when delivered under near ideal circumstances. Efficacy is usually determined by a randomized controlled trial.

Efficiency. The effects or outcomes achieved compared to the resources (e.g. money, staff and time) utilized. It can also be used as a measure of the economy with which a procedure or intervention with a known efficacy is implemented.

Endemic. The constant presence of a disease or infectious agent in a given population or geographical area. Also used to refer to a disease with a near constant incidence of new cases in the area.

Epidemic. The occurrence in a community or region of cases of an illness or other similar event clearly in excess of what is normally expected. The characteristics of the illness, the area and the season all have to be taken into account. To judge whether there is an excess of cases or not requires knowledge about the previous incidence of the event in the same area.

Epidemiology. The study of the distribution and determinants of health and disease in populations and its application to the prevention and control of health problems and diseases.

Eradication. The extermination of an infectious agent, thus halting transmission of infection such as smallpox which has been eradicated throughout the world and dracunculiaisis and polio which are close to being eradicated.

Error. A false or mistaken result obtained in a study or experiment. Errors may be random, in which case they may be disregarded, or systematic, in which case results or findings are biased in one direction.

Evaluation. A process that attempts to determine as systematically and objectively as possible the relevance, effectiveness, and impact of activities in the light of their objectives. Evaluation is often carried out separately for inputs, processes, outcomes, and impact.

Expectation of life (syn: life expectancy). The average time, expressed as the number of years, an individual is expected to live if current mortality trends continue. Life expectancy at birth is the average number of years a newborn can be expected to live under current conditions. Since many deaths in developing countries occur during infancy and childhood, the average life expectancy at birth in these countries is much lower than in developed countries.

Exposure. Often used to define a group exposed to a particular cause of disease or agent as a determinant of health status.

F

False negative. A false result in a screening test, leading to the erroneous classification of a person who is actually positive as a 'negative' or being disease-free.

False positive. The occurrence of a positive test result in a subject who is actually negative, by which a healthy person is wrongly said to have a particular disease or attribute.

Fertility rate. See General fertility rate.

Foetal death rate. Also called stillbirth rate. The number of foetal deaths in one year expressed as a proportion of all births (live plus stillbirths) in the same year. Foetal deaths are deaths prior to the complete expulsion or extraction from its mother of a product of conception. Defined variously as death after the 20th or 28th week of gestation.

Foetal death rate

$$= \frac{\text{No. of foetal deaths in one year}}{\text{No. of foetal deaths plus total live births in same year}} \times 1{,}000$$

Focus group. Small sample of people brought together in order to discuss a topic or issue to ascertain the range and intensity of views or explanations. Often used to explore health-related perceptions and meanings or test out questionnaires.

G

General fertility rate. Similar to the crude birth rate, except that the denominator is restricted to women of childbearing age, that is 15–44 or 15–49 years.

General fertility rate

$$= \frac{\text{No. of live births in a given area in one year}}{\text{Average female population aged } 15 - 44 \text{ years for same area and same year}} \times 1{,}000$$

Geographical information system. Digitally constructed maps using coordinates based on satellites and remote sensing and using sophisticated modelling techniques to analyse data.

Global burden of disease. Indication of the loss of healthy life years from disease around the world, based on DALYs.

Growth rate of populations. Also known as the natural rate of population increase. In the absence of the effects of migration, it is calculated as the difference between crude birth rate and crude death rate, expressed as a percentage.

H

Health. According to the Constitution of the World Health Organization (WHO) (1948), a state of complete physical, mental, and social well-being and not merely the absence of disease or infirmity.

Health behaviour. The combination of knowledge, attitudes, and practices that contribute to the actions taken for health. Behaviours may promote good health, for example healthy eating and compliance with vaccination, or be a determinant by leading to harmful effects, such as may follow smoking and alcohol consumption.

Health equity. Achieving fairness and impartiality in health outcomes and the elimination of unfair and remediable differences among different groups in the population. It is particularly concerned with achieving equity of access to health services and public health programmes regardless of social, ethnic, and cultural status.

Health indicator. A measure that reflects, or indicates, the state of health of persons in a defined population, for example the infant mortality rate or the prevalence of overweight.

Health information system. A combination of health statistics from various sources, used to derive information about health status, health care, provision and use of services, and impact on health.

Herd immunity. The resistance of a group or community to invasion and spread of an infectious agent, due to the resistance to infection in a high proportion of individual members of the group. The herd immunity results in the lowered probability of the disease agent being transmitted from an infected person to a susceptible one when a high proportion of individuals are not susceptible. Also known as population immunity.

Holoendemic. Describes a disease that is virtually universal in the population, with symptoms in childhood, leading to a state of equilibrium and a lower incidence of symptoms in adults, for example malaria in some communities.

Host. A person or animal that is infected under natural conditions. Some microorganisms and parasites may have several different hosts.

Household survey. The collection of information from a representative sample of households by trained interviewers using questionnaires. It is usually a cross-sectional survey to collect information about individual members and on common features, for example water supply and diets.

Hyperendemic. A disease that is constantly present at a high incidence (or prevalence) and that affects all age groups, for example malaria in parts of the African continent.

I

Immunization. The artificial induction of active immunity. Protection of susceptible individuals from communicable disease by administration of a living or modified agent (as in yellow fever), a suspension of killed organisms (as in whooping cough), an inactivated toxin (as in tetanus), or the more recently developed 'subunit, recombinant, polysaccharide, and conjugate vaccines' that use specific pieces of the germ such as its protein, sugar, or capsid (a casing around the germ).

Incidence. The number of instances of new illness commencing, or of persons falling ill, during a given period in a specified population. More generally, the number of new health-related events in a defined population within a specified period of time. It may be measured as a frequency count, a rate, or a proportion. See Incidence rate, Cumulative incidence.

Incidence rate. A measure of the rate at which new cases or events occur in a defined population, also known as incidence density. The numerator is the number of new events, for example new cases of an illness, that occur in a defined period. The denominator is the population at risk of experiencing the event during this period, sometimes expressed as person-time (most often, person-years). The incidence rate most often used in public health practice is calculated from the formula below, where the average number of persons is approximated by the mid-year population in the geographic area of interest.

$$\frac{\text{Number of new events in specified period}}{\text{Average number of persons exposed to risk during this period}} \times 10^n$$

Incubation period. The time interval between the invasion of a susceptible host by an infectious agent and the appearance of the first symptom or sign of the disease, most often expressed as a range of numbers of days. For example, the incubation period of Covid-19 is on average 5–6 days but can be as long as 14 days.

Index case. First case in a group to come to the attention of the investigator, such as in a disease outbreak.

Infant mortality rate. A measure of the yearly rate at which deaths occur in children less than one year old.

$$\text{Infant mortality rate} = \frac{\text{Number of deaths in children less than 1 year old in one year}}{\text{Number of live births in same year}} \times 1{,}000$$

The denominator is an approximation of the total population at risk. This is often used as an indicator of the level of health in a community. Strictly speaking this is a ratio as it is based on infant deaths occurring in a calendar year (including deaths of infants born in the preceding year) over live births in the same calendar year, including births of children who may die in infancy during the next calendar year.

M

Maternal mortality ratio. A measure of a woman's risk of dying from causes associated with childbirth. A maternal death is the death of a woman while pregnant or within 42 days of the termination of pregnancy, irrespective of the duration and the site of pregnancy, from any cause related to or aggravated by the pregnancy or its management, but not from accidental or incidental causes. Some countries have extended the period of 42 days to 1 year.

Maternal deaths are subdivided into direct (e.g. due to haemorrhage or eclampsia) or indirect obstetric deaths resulting from pre-existing disease or disease that developed during pregnancy and was not due to direct obstetric causes, but which was aggravated by a physiological effects of pregnancy. The death of a pregnant woman from an incidental cause (e.g. motor car accident) is not classified as a maternal death.

Maternal mortality ratio

$$= \frac{\text{Number of maternal deaths in given area in one year}}{\text{Number of live births in the same area during the same year}} \times 1,000$$

Mean, arithmetic. This is also commonly called the average. It is calculated by adding together all the individual values in a set of measurements and dividing this total by the number of values in the set.

Measurement scale. The complete range of possible values for a measurement (e.g. the set of possible responses to a question, the possible range for a set of body weights). Scales can be divided into five main types:

Dichotomous: two mutually exclusive groups, for example positive and negative
Nominal: qualitative categories, for example for religions
Ordinal: ordered qualitative categories, for example social classes I to V
Interval: scale with equal distances for each interval but no particular starting or zero point, for example date of birth
Ratio: interval scale with a zero starting point, for example weight, blood pressure, income

Median. The central value in a range of measurements that divides the set into two equal parts.

Mode. The most frequently occurring value in a set of observations.

Monitoring. The continuous measurement and observation of changes in the health status of populations or in the physical or social environment. In the context of a service or programme, monitoring is essential to see that it is proceeding according to the proposed plans and objectives. In management, monitoring includes the episodic oversight of the implementation of an activity, seeking to ensure that input deliveries, work schedules, targeted outputs, and other required actions are proceeding according to plan. If monitoring reveals that there are problems, management decisions will have to be taken to alter or improve the service or programme so that it comes back on track.

Morbidity. Any departure from a state of physiological or psychological well-being. Morbidity can be expressed in terms of people who are ill, episodes of illness, and/or the duration of these illnesses. All morbidity statistics must refer to the number of people being monitored and the corresponding time period.

N

Neonatal mortality rate. The number of deaths in infants under 28 days of age in a given period, usually one year, per 1,000 live births in the same period.

Non-respondents. Members of a study sample or population who, for whatever reason, do not respond or do not take part in the study. Respondents may differ from non-respondents and a high non-response rate may be an important source of bias.

Notifiable disease. A disease that, by statutory requirements, must be reported to the public health authority in the pertinent jurisdiction when the diagnosis is made. The disease is deemed of sufficient importance to the public health to require that its occurrence be reported to health authorities.

Numerator. The upper portion of a fraction, used to calculate a rate or a ratio.

O

Observational study. Study, survey, or investigation made by observing subjects and where no interventions are implemented at the same time. Most analytical epidemiological designs (e.g. case-control, cross-sectional, and cohort studies) are properly called observational because investigators observe without any interventions other than to record, classify, count, and statistically analyse results. Many important epidemiological, clinical, and microbiological studies are completely observational or have large observational components. See also Randomized controlled trials.

Observer variation (error). Variation or error in measurements due to failure of the observer to measure or identify the phenomenon accurately. Variation can be due to such faults as the observer missing an observation, poor technique, incorrect reading or recording, and misinterpretation of answers to questions. Observer error is particularly important if it is non-random and therefore can lead to bias in one direction, for example when an observer is more likely to record sick people as being healthy.

Odds. The ratio of the probability of occurrence of an event to that of nonoccurrence. For example if 20% of subjects examined are hypertensive and 80% are normal, the odds of hypertension is equal to 20 divided by 80, or 25%; this may be contrasted with the prevalence or probability of hypertension, which is 20 over 100 or 20%. Ratios are always larger than the corresponding probability, particularly for common health outcomes.

In the case of a disease (e.g. hypertension) this is referred to as disease odds. For a risk factor, such as smoking, this referred to exposure odds. For example, if 30% of the sample are smokers the exposure odds will be equal to 30 over 70, or 43%.

Odds ratio. The ratio of two odds, such as exposure odds as in case-control or cross-sectional study, or disease odds in a cohort study.

Output. The immediate results of professional or institutional health care activities, expressed as units of service (e.g. patient hospital days, out-patient visits, laboratory tests performed, vaccines administered).

P

P or probability value. The letter *P* followed by <, the symbol for less than, and a number (usually 0.05, 0.01, or 0.001) is a statement of the probability that the association or observation under investigation could have occurred by chance. The number 0.05 means the observation would be expected to occur by chance 1 in 20 times; similarly, 0.01 means 1 in 100. An association is commonly accepted as statistically significant if *P* is < 0.05. *P* followed by *n.s.* indicates that the observation is not significant at the level chosen.

Pandemic. An epidemic occurring worldwide or over a very wide area, crossing international boundaries, and usually affecting a large number of people. As in the case of Covid-19, presence of a pandemic must be declared by the World Health Organization.

Pathogenesis. The mechanism by which a cause or etiological agent produces disease. The aetiology of a disease, disability or other health state begins with causes that initiate pathogenesis or favor pathogenetic mechanisms; control of such causes favours primary prevention of the disease.

Percentile. Set of divisions that produces 100 equal parts for a continuous variable, for example weight. Thus, a child above the 90th percentile has a greater value for height or weight than over 90% of all in the series. Percentiles are often divided into quintiles (five groups, each of which with 20% of all observations) or deciles (ten groups, each with 10%).

Perinatal mortality rate. The officially accepted definition is as follows:

$$\frac{\text{Late foetal deaths}\ (28\ \text{weeks or more}\ )+1^{st}-\text{week postnatal deaths}}{\text{All births (late foetal deaths plus total births)},\ \text{same population \& period}}\times 1{,}000$$

Some countries with inadequate vital statistics do not include foetal deaths in the denominator, and express it as a rate per 1,000 live births per year. When gestational age cannot be adequately measured, as in many low-income countries, the alternative definition is 'late foetal and early neonatal deaths weighing over 1000 g at birth expressed as a ratio per 1000 live births weighing over 1000 g at birth'.

The perinatal mortality rate is a useful indicator for the quality of antenatal, obstetric, and newborn care.

Person-time. A measurement combining persons and time as the denominator in incidence and mortality rates, when for varying periods individuals are at risk of developing disease or dying. It is the sum of all the periods of time at risk for each of the subjects. The most widely used measure is person-years.

With this approach, each subject contributes only as many years of observation to the population at risk as the period over which that subject has been observed to be at risk of the disease; a subject observed over 1 year contributes 1 person-year, a subject observed over a 10-year period contributes 10 person-years. This method can be used to measure an incidence rate over extended and variable time periods.

Population. The total number of inhabitants of a given area or country. In sampling, the population may refer to the units from which the sample is drawn, not necessarily the total population of people. The term population is also commonly also used to refer to particular priority or high-risk groups.

Population pyramid. A graphical representation of the age and sex composition of a population. This is constructed by computing the percentage distribution (or absolute numbers) of a population when cross-classified by sex and age. The percentage that each female age group represents in the total population is plotted on the right and the corresponding percentages for males are on the left. A pyramid with a broad base, sloping sides, and narrow apex is typical of many developing countries. This shape is due to high fertility and high mortality at younger ages.

Post-neonatal mortality rate. The number of infant deaths between 28 days and one year of age in a given year per 1,000 live births in that year. In low- and middle-income countries this rate largely reflects deaths due to infectious diseases and malnutrition.

Predictive value. The probability that a person with a positive (or negative) result in a screening or diagnostic test is in fact a true positive (or true negative). These are called the positive and negative predictive values of the test. The predictive value depends on the sensitivity and specificity of the test and on the prevalence of the condition being screened. See Validity and Annex Four.

Prevalence. The number of cases or events or conditions in a given population at a particular point in time (known as point prevalence), divided by the population at risk of having the disease, event, or condition. Period prevalence refers to cases or events at any time during a given period; for example, annual prevalence includes cases of the disease arising before but extending into or through the year, as well as those having their inception during the year, and also those who present the condition at a certain time during the year but have recovered. Prevalence measures are mostly suited for diseases or events that have long average duration, for example hypertension or diabetes. Prevalence measures are proportions, not rates, although the expression 'prevalence rate' is often used. See Rate.

Prevalence study or survey. See Cross-sectional study.

Prevention. Measures aimed at promoting and maintaining health, with such interventions as improving nutritional status, immunization, suitable water supplies, and excreta disposal (primary prevention). Secondary prevention comprises measures aimed at ensuring the early detection of diseases and infections, whereas tertiary prevention is concerned with reducing symptomatic illness and disability.

Q

Qualitative research. Research that uses non-numerical methods to explore individual and group characteristics with findings that are not usually subject to statistical analysis or other quantitative means. Examples include clinical case descriptions, narrative studies of behaviour, ethnography, and organizational or social studies. Methods include observation, review of documents, key informant interviews, and focus group discussions.

Quality assurance. A system of procedures, checks, audits, and corrective actions to ensure that all procedures, research activities, and programmes achieve the highest quality possible.

Quarantine. Restriction of the activities of persons or animals who have been exposed to cases of communicable diseases during its period of communicability (i.e. contacts) to prevent further transmission during the incubation period when infection might occur.

R

Random. Describes a happening or event due to chance and not determined by other factors.

Random allocation, randomization. The separation or allocation of individuals or groups of individuals to two or more groups at random. Within the limits of chance variation (e.g. if the number of subjects is large), it yields groups similar at the start of an investigation for both known and unknown variables (i.e. including measured and unmeasured determinants of the outcomes). No other methodological procedure can accomplish this.

Randomized controlled trial. An experiment where participants or groups of participants are randomly allocated to intervention (treatment) groups or to a control group. The results are assessed by looking for any significant difference between these groups. These trials are the most rigorous and scientific way of testing the efficacy of new interventions. They can, however, lack generalizability if the sample of participants is not representative of people or patients in the specific population for whom the intervention is intended. This can also be due to too many participants being ineligible or refusing to take part.

Random sample. A sample derived by random selection of sample units. Each unit, for example a person, household, or village, should have an equal chance of being included in the sample. When the chance of being included is not equal for all units, weighting is required in the analysis phase to reproduce the original population.

Rate. A measure of the frequency with which an event occurs in a defined population within a specified period of time. The rate is composed of the numerator, denominator, specified time period, and the multiplying factor, for example 100 or 1,000. In vital statistics the denominator is usually the average population during a one-year period, or the estimated mid-year population. In epidemiological studies such as cohorts, the person-time denominator can be calculated from information on the date of recruitment and the date when individuals either suffered the event (illness onset or death) or were lost to follow-up.

The use of rates rather than raw numbers is essential for comparison of experience between populations at different times, different places, or among different classes of persons.

Register. A file of data concerning all cases of disease or a health event in a defined population. From this register cases can be followed up, and incidence, prevalence, and survival can be calculated. Examples are cancer, tuberculosis, and pregnancy registries.

Relative risk. The ratio of the risk of death or disease in an exposed population to the risk in the unexposed population. Strictly speaking, a relative risk is the ratio of cumulative incidence (or risk) among the exposed to cumulative incidence among the unexposed. The term is widely used also for odds ratios, for ratios of incidence densities (or rate ratios), and for prevalence ratios.

Repeatability. The ability of a test to produce results that are identical or closely similar each time it is conducted. Precision is another term that is often used. Reliability is the degree to which a measurement can be replicated. See also Accuracy and Validity.

Representative sample. A sample that resembles the original population or reference population in accordance to measurable characteristics. To ensure this, all samples should be selected by random methods and then compared with the original population for important variables, for example age and sex.

Reproductive rate. Also referred to as the basic reproductive rate, or the R0 (R zero) parameter. A measure of the number of infections produced, on average, by an infected individual in the early stages of an epidemic when nearly all contacts are susceptible. See Attack rate and Secondary attack rate.

Reservoir of infection. The natural habitat of an infectious agent, which may be a person, animal, arthropod, plant, soil, etc. It is where the agent normally lives and multiplies.

Response rate. The number of interviews or examinations completed divided by the total due to have been carried out, expressed as a percentage. High non-response rates can be an important source of bias. Usually expressed as a percentage.

Retrospective study. A research design used to test etiological hypotheses in which inferences about exposure to the putative causal factor(s) are derived from data relating to characteristics of the persons under study or to events or experiences in their past. The essential feature is that some of the persons under study have the disease or other outcome condition of interest, and their characteristics and past experiences are compared with those of other, unaffected persons. The term 'retrospective study' used to be a synonym for a case-control study, but other study designs may also be retrospective such as retrospective cohort studies.

Risk. The probability that an event will occur, for example that an individual will become ill or die within a stated period of time or at/by a given age. The term is usually used with reference to unfavourable events. The strict definition of risk is the same as that of cumulative incidence. See Cumulative Incidence.

Risk factor. The term is used in at least two different ways. First as an attribute, variable, or exposure that is associated with an increased probability of a subsequent specified event, for example the occurrence of a disease. These preceding factors are not necessarily causal and are often called risk markers. Secondly, an attribute, variable, or exposure that actually increases the occurrence of a specified event and is therefore believed to be causal (also described as a determinant).

S

Sample. A selected subset of a population. A sample may be random or non-random and it may be representative or non-representative. In an *epsem* (equal probability of selection method) sample all the population units have an equal chance of being selected. A simple random sample of individuals is an *epsem* sample.

Random samples may also be selected with different probabilities of selection, for example rural areas may be oversampled; when this occurs, the resulting estimates need to be weighted to reproduce the total population, and the sample is described as a stratified sample. See Representativeness.

Scattergram Using dots displaying the distribution between two variables on the horizontal axis and vertical axis.

Screening. The presumptive identification of previously unrecognized disease or behaviour or marker by using tests, examinations, questionnaires, and other procedures. Screening sorts people into positives and negatives. People who are positive will probably require further investigation. It is important to examine the results for the proportion of false positives and false negatives. A screening test is not necessarily intended to be diagnostic. See also Sensitivity and Specificity and Annex Four.

Secondary attack rate. The number of new cases that occur (within the accepted incubation period of the disease) among contacts of a primary or earlier case, divided by the number of exposed for contact. The secondary attack rate is a measure of contagiousness and is useful in evaluating control measures. See Attack rate and Reproductive rate.

Sensitivity. The proportion of true positives correctly identified by a screening test, or the probability that a diseased person (or case) in the population tested will be identified as diseased by the test. See Predictive Value and Specificity, and Annex Four.

Sero-epidemiology. The use of serological investigations, particularly antibody levels, to detect infection and transmission patterns. Latent, sub-clinical infections and carrier states may be detected in addition to the clinically overt cases.

Socioeconomic status or socioeconomic position. A descriptive classification of a person's position in society, using such criteria as household assets, income, educational level, occupation, and dwelling place. Attitudes towards health, use of services, and health status are often closely linked to socioeconomic status. See Asset index.

Specificity. The proportion of true negatives correctly identified by a screening test. See also Predictive value and Sensitivity.

Sporadic. A disease or event that occurs infrequently and irregularly. A term usually applied to certain communicable diseases.

Spot map. A map showing the geographical distribution of people with a particular characteristic, commonly used in the investigation and control of an epidemic.

Standard deviation. A measure of the dispersion or variation of a set of quantitative observations or measurements on either side of the mean or average. It is equal to the positive square root of the variance.

Standardization. Application of statistical techniques to standardize two or more populations for differences that may exist among them, particularly as regards age and sex population structure to enable valid comparisons to be made. Further information is available in Annex One.

Standardized mortality ratio (SMR). The ratio of the number of deaths observed in the study population compared to the number that would be expected if the study population had the same mortality rate as the general population, expressed as a percentage.

Statistical significance. See *P* or Probability value.

Stillbirth rate. See Foetal death rate.

Surveillance. The process of systematic and continuous collection, orderly consolidation, and evaluation of pertinent data with timely dissemination of the results to those who need to know, in particular those who are in a position to take action. Surveillance is essential in disease control and in the monitoring of programme effectiveness.

Susceptibility. Lack of immunity or weak resistance to a disease, usually referring to an agent causing a communicable disease. This can result in an exposure being more likely to lead to a sub-clinical or clinical infection.

T

Target. A desired programme outcome that is explicitly stated, for example coverage to be achieved for immunization or treatment of tuberculosis cases. A target usually includes a stated time frame. The Sustainable Development Goals include several specific targets that countries have subscribed to and aim to achieve to improve global health by 2030.

Total fertility rate. An estimate of the average number of children that would be born per woman if all women lived to the end of their childbearing years and bore children according to current age-specific fertility rates. It provides an answer to the question: How many children does a woman have on average during her lifetime?

Transmission of infection. The spread of an infectious agent, either through the environment or from person to person. The main mechanisms of transmission are: direct contact, placental, droplets, dust, foodborne, waterborne, airborne (aerosols), and vector-borne.

Trend. A long-term general movement or change in frequency over time, usually either upward or downward. A downward trend in a disease or unhealthy behaviour means that it is becoming less frequent. Another definition of trend refers to an association that is consistent in several samples or strata but is not statistically significant.

U, V, W, X, Y, Z

Underlying cause of death. The disease or injury that initiated the series of events leading directly to death or the circumstances of the accident or violence that produced the fatal injury.

Under-reporting. Failure to identify or count all cases or events, leading to a numerator that is smaller than the true one. This leads to estimates of frequency that are lower than the true value.

Validity. The degree to which a measurement actually measures or detects what it is supposed to measure. This concept is particularly important in screening procedures. See Accuracy and Repeatability.

Variable. Any measurable characteristic or attribute that can assume different values.

Virulence. The degree of pathogenicity, or ability to produce disease, of an infectious agent. Numerically expressed as the ratio of the number of cases of overt infection to the total number infected as determined by laboratory tests. When death is the only criterion of severity, this is the case-fatality rate.

Vital statistics. Systematically tabulated information about births, marriages, divorces, and deaths, based on registration of these vital events.

Zero reporting. The reporting of 'zero cases' is when no cases have been detected by the reporting unit. This allows the next level of the reporting system to be sure that the participant has not sent data that have been lost or that the participant has not forgotten to report.

Zoonosis. An infectious or communicable disease that can be transmitted from vertebrate animals to human beings. Examples include rabies and plague. May be enzootic or epizootic.

Useful Publications

Abramson JH and Abramson ZH. *Research Methods in Community Medicine—Surveys, Epidemiological Research, Programme Evaluation, and Clinical Trials*, 6th edn (Wiley, 2008).

American Public Health Association. *Control of Communicable Diseases Manual*, 20th edn (Washington, DC: APHA Press, 2015).

Barry JM. *The Great Influenza* (London: Penguin, 2018).

Bonita R, Beaglehole R, and Kjellstrom T. *Basic Epidemiology*, 2nd edn (Geneva: World Health Organization, 2006) available for free from WHO Geneva in several languages, <https://apps.who.int/iris/bitstream/handle/10665/43541/9241547073_eng.pdf?sequence=1&isAllowed=y>

Persson LA and Wall S. *Epidemiology for Public Health* (Umea, Sweden: Department of Public Health and Clinical Medicine, 2000).

Porter M (ed). *A Dictionary of Epidemiology*, 6th edn (Oxford: Oxford University Press, 2014).

Rogers A and Vaughan JP. *World Health Report 2002: Reducing Risks, Promoting Health Life.* C Murray and A Lopez overall direction; (Geneva: World Health Organization, 2002).

Rose G. *Strategy of Preventive Medicine* (Oxford: Oxford University Press, 2008).

Scrimshaw SCM and Hurtado E. Rapid assessment procedures for nutrition and primary health care: anthropological approaches to improving programme effectiveness. 1989.

Siegel JS. *The Demography and Epidemiology of Human Health and Aging* (Amsterdam: Springer Netherlands, 2012).

Smith PG, Morrow RH, and Ross DA (eds). *Field Trials of Health Interventions—A Tool Box*, 3rd edn (Oxford: Oxford University Press, 2015), available for free at: https://ieaweb.org/docs/Field-trials-of-health-interventions-a-toolbox-with-full-hyperlinks-July-15.pdf

Vaughan JP and Morrow RH. *Manual of Epidemiology for District Health Management* (Geneva: World Health Organization, 1989), available for free from WHO in several languages.

Whitehead M. 'The concepts and principles of equity and health' (1992) 22(3) International Journal of Health Services 429–45. doi: 10.2190/986L-LHQ6-2VTE-YRRN.

World Bank. *Handbook on Impact Evaluation: Quantitative Methods and Practices* (Washington, DC: World Bank, 2010) <https://openknowledge.worldbank.org/handle/10986/2693>

On Sustainable Development Goals related to health <www.un.org/sustainabledevelopment>

On Universal Health Coverage <www.who.int/uhc>

For comments on Universal Health Coverage <https://www.thelancet.com/journals/lancet/article/PIIS0140-6736(19)31831-8/fulltext>

For analysis and use of health facility data <https://www.who.int/healthinfo/tools_data_analysis_routinefacilities/en/>

For EpiInfo version 7 menu and user guide <https://www.cdc.gov/epiinfo/support/userguide.html>

ANNEXES

ANNEX ONE

Population Standardization

Incorrect conclusions can also be avoided by using age-specific rates or age standardization. Age standardization is based on using weighted averaging to remove possible differences when comparing two or more populations due to their age or sex or structure or any other related confounding variables. It is used to adjust rates and other measures for any age and sex differences between two or more populations.

Using Age- and Sex-specific Rates

These are separate rates that are specific for men and women and for specific age groups. The numerator and denominator both refer to the same age and sex specific groups. Comparing age- and sex-specific rates is essential before carrying out standardization procedures. Any unusual findings in such rates should be investigated for potential data errors or unusual characteristics in the population.

Using Direct Age and Sex Standardization

The specific rates in a study population are averaged by using as weights the distribution of a specified standard population. The standardized rate represents what the crude rate would have been in the study population if it had the same distribution as the standard population with respect to both age and sex.

Using EpiInfo

Statistical software such as EpiInfo is a useful tool for standardization. Standardization can also easily be performed using a spreadsheet program such as Excel.

Example: Comparing prevalence rates in two Villages A and B for age differences

Two villages, endemic for schistosomiasis, each have a population of 500 who were examined for the presence of *Schistosomiasis mansoni* eggs in faecal specimens. The two villages were thought to be similar for their total population, age range, and male to female sex ratio. The overall prevalence rates for the total populations in villages A and B are shown in the table below:

Comparison of crude prevalence rate of *Schistosoma mansoni* infection in Villages A and B

Age (years)	Village A			Village B			Standard population (A + B)
	No. examined	No. positive	% positive	No. examined	No. positive	% positive	
0–4	50	5	10	50	5	10	100
5–9	100	40	40	50	20	40	150
10–14	150	120	80	50	40	80	200
15–19	80	56	70	80	56	70	160
20–29	70	21	30	120	36	30	190
30+	50	10	20	150	30	20	200
TOTAL	500	252	50.4	500	187	37.4	1,000

Reproduced with permission from Vaughan, J Patrick, Morrow, Richard H, and World Health Organization, Manual of epidemiology for district health management, World Health Organization; Geneva, Switzerland, Copyright © 1989

$$\text{The difference between the two rates} = \frac{50.4 - 37.4}{\text{Standard error}} = 4.2 \; p \text{ less than } 0.01$$

With p less than 0.01 this difference was seen as statistically significant and that there was a true difference in schistosomiasis prevalence rates and that village A was more heavily infected than village B.

While the total prevalence percentage rates were apparently significantly different, all the age specific rates were the same in both villages—see the third column for each village. If the age-specific rates had been used instead then the conclusion would have been different.

The analysis had not standardised for differences in the age structure of the two populations. More people in village A were in the 10–14 years group and this led to a higher rate for the total percentage.

Using direct age standardization

There are four main steps in the analysis:

1. Calculate the prevalence or incidence rates for each group

$$\text{For Example for } 0-4 \text{ year olds in Village A prevalence} = \frac{5 \times 100}{50} = 10\%$$

2. Form a new standard population for each group by adding together A + B
   See last column in the table
3. Age specific rates for A and B are multiplied by the standard population to give the expected total number of infected people in that age group

$$\text{For } 10-14 \text{ year old children the number is} = \frac{80 \times 200}{100} = 160$$

4. If this process is completed for each age group and for each village it will be found that, given the standard age structure, there would be an expected 439 cases

$$\text{Prevalence} = \frac{\text{Total expected cases}}{\text{Total standard population}} \times 100$$

$$= \frac{439}{1,000} \times 100 = 43.9\%$$

Conclusion

Despite the original significance of the p level after standardization there was in fact no significant difference between villages A and B and the original conclusion was therefore incorrect. The apparent difference had not taken into account that the two villages did indeed have different age structures.

The reverse conclusion can also happen when an apparently insignificant difference can become statistically significant after standardization although this is less common.

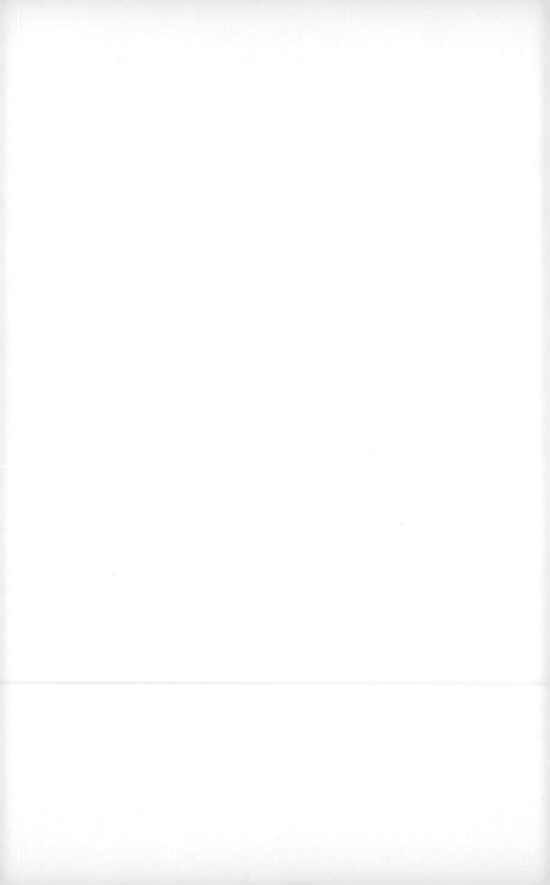

Using Random Numbers

To draw a random sample for a study population, the random numbers table below can be used. For a reference population in 130 listed villages and a required random cluster sample of 10 villages:

1. As the reference population lives in 130 villages (three figures), select any 3 adjacent single number columns between 1 and 40, say columns 11, 12, and 13
2. Run down these columns to select the first 10 numbers between 1 and 130, say 48, 81, and 72, etc.
3. At the end of columns 11, 12, and 13 start again with the next 3 columns, say 14, 15, and 16
4. Proceed until 10 numbers are selected, which correspond to the village numbers in the listing
5. Randomly select 10 to 20 people from each village or to select a more specific sample such as children aged 0–4 years, or all women 15–44 years old, or adults 15 years or older

For users of Excel, the function RANDBETWEEN(0,130) may be pasted in 10 cells, and each will yield a random number that may then be used for sampling 10 out of 130 units.

1				10	11				20	21				30	31				40
18	10	49	89	75	57	96	23	76	80	93	00	28	92	31	44	33	49	42	80
50	89	75	71	55	27	63	29	98	47	38	94	60	09	62	61	42	86	50	58
11	15	50	84	49	34	67	34	36	82	53	90	49	23	88	06	89	27	08	16
70	25	51	01	81	16	19	30	09	68	02	21	05	62	33	45	95	87	67	47
62	86	38	01	20	04	82	62	77	31	49	63	64	70	99	39	66	55	18	11
95	19	70	36	92	85	05	39	25	78	84	34	14	28	76	20	20	17	79	94
85	61	50	19	61	87	14	59	61	75	53	44	19	12	00	65	02	00	70	99
83	55	66	76	74	68	47	68	66	86	49	47	63	51	43	87	42	58	36	04
90	51	34	31	18	74	55	41	42	81	70	15	36	55	16	10	88	62	68	72
99	56	78	99	98	77	87	25	77	60	34	13	82	02	11	32	31	43	48	10
27	24	80	09	77	14	13	96	19	16	22	48	88	26	25	42	67	93	74	00
34	63	66	89	97	29	99	91	27	17	14	56	41	05	32	90	14	45	30	61
28	98	45	23	35	60	68	32	66	37	43	44	27	92	07	91	64	22	32	72
06	96	34	21	67	08	12	58	74	35	91	64	68	15	01	36	52	07	00	39
19	62	94	14	54	83	15	22	30	16	92	99	79	27	67	13	22	25	43	19
44	36	96	82	39	55	96	96	89	04	43	89	96	59	17	10	84	24	12	44
76	96	59	93	98	79	41	35	91	77	66	88	50	31	77	06	24	08	19	51
31	61	97	08	88	35	43	85	84	51	94	85	55	05	33	86	42	20	51	41
42	95	12	75	72	33	23	70	66	71	76	89	28	45	92	12	21	41	92	53
95	42	30	03	62	83	35	78	07	35	67	85	83	57	36	96	97	62	67	06
48	55	12	87	21	41	86	33	99	44	83	14	01	42	54	59	31	64	10	04
46	18	81	87	56	81	03	74	48	49	28	37	85	93	69	84	92	33	52	70
66	47	43	88	02	61	25	59	10	35	09	65	92	36	93	47	04	89	17	03
61	91	88	50	00	19	31	08	80	39	14	03	80	46	41	78	82	03	69	52
85	74	04	57	53	44	43	44	61	57	29	24	36	38	79	49	25	39	73	02
89	09	53	94	07	92	21	54	01	70	31	91	39	51	03	94	83	98	31	15
54	87	27	50	35	73	27	60	10	55	13	21	24	10	55	84	78	88	46	83
49	13	89	98	96	21	02	44	94	30	50	70	71	02	16	35	31	13	14	45
97	37	11	88	77	45	16	03	17	01	00	67	28	09	39	28	39	11	36	82
99	70	37	54	02	40	71	13	59	37	84	38	47	11	31	48	92	28	96	37
65	67	36	23	39	07	20	59	36	85	47	17	51	32	75	07	74	63	68	01
53	69	94	34	45	46	09	52	84	40	82	80	75	72	79	43	97	07	96	15
54	08	33	44	54	42	81	46	46	42	01	44	13	13	97	35	11	85	48	41
95	54	39	60	78	27	35	07	35	53	93	29	83	01	86	52	11	41	68	50
88	79	66	20	03	48	81	94	46	07	91	39	12	45	51	68	94	53	77	83
68	82	57	41	23	57	52	47	09	83	11	27	88	40	16	22	64	86	22	18
55	73	62	41	71	45	35	51	28	64	82	46	10	85	71	21	57	92	10	58
17	50	60	03	20	35	64	36	90	97	29	78	17	83	29	08	99	20	47	79
11	54	11	75	35	76	49	67	96	84	11	75	73	34	90	97	74	85	88	37
78	32	11	34	33	55	30	20	68	10	68	96	94	82	04	94	10	52	73	51

Sample Size for Prevalence Surveys

If the sample is correctly selected, the larger it is the closer the estimate of prevalence is likely to be to the true prevalence in the whole community. A smaller sample will require less time and costs, and quality control and supervision will ensure better accuracy and repeatability of the data collected.

The required sample size is the smallest one that will give an acceptable level of accuracy. The table below shows the minimum sample sizes for various levels of expected prevalence and specified margins of sampling error for the estimated prevalence.

To use this table first select the appropriate column according to how close to 50% the prevalence is expected to be. If the figure is higher than 50% then use 100 minus this figure. Next select a row in the table according to the amount of sampling error that can be tolerated for the estimated rate.

For example, if it is suspected that the prevalence of schistosomiasis is between 20% and 40% and that the survey should have a good chance of estimating the prevalence to within 5% points of its true value, a random sample of at least 369 is necessary. If the survey sample shows a prevalence of 32.5% the prevalence range is 32.5%, plus or minus 5% points, that is between 27.5% and 37.5%.

Margin of sampling error tolerated[1]	Maximum expected prevalence rate (%)[2]							
	1%	2.5%	5%	10%	20%	30%	40%	50%
0.5%	1 522	3,746	7,300	13,830	—	—	—	—
1%	381	937	1,825	3,458	6,147	8,068	9,220	9,604
2%	—	235	457	865	1,537	2,017	2,305	2,401
5%	—	—	73	139	246	323	369	385
10%	—	—	—	35	62	81	93	97
15%	—	—	—	—	28	36	41	43

[1] This represents the 95% confidence interval. For example, if the true prevalence was 10% and we took a sample of size 139 we would be 95% certain that the prevalence measured in the sample would be between 5% and 15% (i.e. 10 ± 5%). In general, do not accept a sampling error of greater than 5%.
[2] Select the highest rate that the prevalence is likely to be. If the rate is expected to be higher than 50%, use 100 minus the expected rate.

Reproduced with permission from Vaughan, J Patrick, Morrow, Richard H, and World Health Organization, Manual of epidemiology for district health management, World Health Organization; Geneva, Switzerland, Copyright © 1989

The sampling error tolerated is for a 95% confidence interval. If the true prevalence was 10% and the sample size was 139, we would be 95% certain that prevalence in this sample would be between 5% and 15%, that is, 10% plus or minus. The maximum acceptable sampling error should not be more than 5% points.

With a low prevalence condition, such as leprosy or tuberculosis, with a prevalence rate of 1–2%, a margin of error of 1% point might be acceptable. A 1% point error on an estimated prevalence of 2.5% would require a sample of at least 937 people. For a reasonable accurate estimate, therefore, the survey sample would need to be about 1,000 people.

When estimating required sample sizes for a study, it is useful to add say 10% for non-response. For example, if the table above shows that you need 90 individuals, we suggest aiming at examining 99 people, that is 90% plus 10% of 90%. If you think non-response will be higher or lower than 10%, you may change the number of additional individuals required.

Screening and Diagnostic Tests

Validity and predictive value

The **validity** and the **predictive** value of screening and diagnostic and tests have to be considered when they are used in surveys, special studies, and as screening tests. For instance, tests may be based on standardized interviews, physical examinations, or laboratory tests, or more sophisticated measurements such as body scans, electrocardiograms, and histopathology.

Validity of tests refers to the extent to which the test is capable of correctly diagnosing the presence or absence of the concerned disease or condition. These two aspects—presence or absence—are referred to as the **sensitivity** and **specificity** of the test. For example, a test has a sensitivity of 90% if it gives a positive result in 90% of people **with** the disease or condition.

A test has a specificity of 90% if it gives a negative result in 90% of people who actually do **not** have the disease or condition.

Estimating the validity of a test requires a comparison with a well-established test or diagnosis for the disease or condition being examined. For example, rapid tests for antibodies against the SARS-CoV-2 virus (the type 2 coronavirus) may be compared to a polymerase chain reaction (PCR) test that is used to confirm the infection. The 'true test' is often referred to as the 'gold standard'.

The test is always compared to the 'true' value, as shown in the table below:

		Test result		
		Positive	Negative	Total
'True' disease	Present	a	b	$a + b$
	Absent	c	d	$c + d$
Total		$a + c$	$b + d$	$a + b + c + d$
Sensitivity		$\dfrac{a}{a+b}$	**Specificity**	$\dfrac{d}{c+d}$
	False negatives =	b	False positives =	c
True prevalence	=	$\dfrac{a+b}{a+b+c+d}$		

True prevalence can only be calculated when a + b + c + d is a representative sample of the population:

$$\textbf{Positive predictive } \text{value of test} = \frac{a}{a+c}$$

$$\textbf{Negative predictive } \text{value of test} = \frac{d}{b+d}$$

Sensitivity and specificity are ratios comparing test results to the 'true' disease or condition. The true overall prevalence of the disease or condition does not affect the sensitivity or specificity of the test, because sensitivity is calculated solely among true positives and specificity among true negatives.

Sensitivity and specificity are proportions comparing test results to the 'true' disease or condition.

However, tests are actually used the other way around when they are needed to predict which individuals have the disease or condition being investigated and hence the importance of using positive and negative 'predictive values'.

Test are usually judged on their sensitivity and specificity. However, the user may also need to make a choice of tests based on their **predictive value**. This is the most important measure for determining its usefulness under 'field' conditions. It depends upon the prevalence of the disease or condition as well as the test's sensitivity and specificity.

The equations below can be used to calculate predictive values for different combinations of disease prevalence and test sensitivity and specificity. These show the relationship between prevalence, sensitivity, specificity, and predictive values:

$$\text{Positive predictive value}(PV+)$$
$$= \frac{\text{Prevalence }(P)\times\text{Sensitivity}}{(\text{Prevalence}\times\text{Sensitivity}+((1-P)\times(1-\text{Specificity})))}$$
$$\text{Negative predictive value}(PV-)$$
$$= \frac{(1-\text{Prevalence})\times\text{Specificity}}{((1-\text{Prevalence})\times\text{Specificity})+(P\times(1-\text{sensitivity}))}$$

How does prevalence affect the positive predictive values?

For example, for a diagnostic test with a sensitivity of 95% used with a condition that has a prevalence of 20%, the positive predictive value for a positive result is 83%, calculated as follows:

$$PV+ = \frac{0.2\times0.95}{(0.2\times0.95)+(0.8\times0.05)} = 0.83 \text{ or } 83\%$$

When the same test is used in a population where the disease prevalence is only 1%, the positive predictive value is only 16%, as follows:

$$PV+ = \frac{0.01\times0.95}{(0.01\times0.95)+(0.99\times0.05)} = 0.16 \text{ or } 16\%$$

This means that of all positives found by the screening test only 16%, or about 1 in 6, are true positives. The reason for this difference is that when prevalence is very low—as in the second example above—most positive subjects according to the test will be represented as false positives.

Predictive value and disease control programmes

This example shows that even with a test with high sensitivity and specificity the positive predictive value will fall from 83% to 16% when the prevalence drops from 20% to 1%. This situation can occur even if a control programme that has been successfully implemented.

For example, in a sample of 2,000 people of known disease status on both occasions, the actual distribution of test results compared to actual disease status is shown in table below. Before the control programme the prevalence rate was 20% with 400 out of 2,000 people with the disease, the test sensitivity and specificity were both 95% and the positive predictive value was 83%.

		Test Result		
		Positive	Negative	Total
Disease present	Yes	380	20	400
	No	80	1520	1600
	Total	460	1,540	2,000

Test sensitivity = 95% (380/400)
Test specificity = 95% (1,520/1,600)
Positive predictive value = 83% (380/460)

Research Ethics and Review of Proposals

CIOMS—Council for International Organizations of Medical Sciences

The CIOMS is an international, non-governmental, non-profit organization established jointly by the World Health Organization (WHO) and the United Nations Educational, Scientific and Cultural Organization (UNESCO) in 1949. The CIOMS mission is to advance public health through guidance on health research and policy including ethics, medical product development, and safety.

CIOMS represents a substantial proportion of the biomedical scientific community through its member organizations, which include many of the biomedical disciplines, national academies of sciences, and medical research councils. CIOMS is in official relations with the WHO and is an associate partner of UNESCO.

Source: www.cioms.ch

What are the basic principles of medical ethics?

Bioethicists often refer to the four basic principles of health care ethics when evaluating the merits and difficulties of medical procedures. Ideally, for a medical study or practice to be considered 'ethical', it must respect all four of the following principles: autonomy, justice, beneficence, and non-maleficence. For instance the use of reproductive technology raises questions in each of these areas.

Autonomy —Requires that patients have autonomy of thought, intention, and action when making decisions regarding health care procedures. The decision-making process must be free of coercion. In order for a patient to make a fully informed decision, she/he must understand all risks and benefits of the procedure(s) and the likelihood of success.

Justice —The idea that the burdens and benefits of new or experimental treatments (or interventions) must be distributed equally among all groups in society. This requires that procedures uphold the spirit of existing laws and are fair to all players involved. The health care provider(s) must consider four main areas when evaluating justice: fair distribution of scarce resources, competing needs, rights and obligations, and potential conflicts with established legislation. For instance, reproductive technologies create ethical dilemmas because treatment is not equally available to all people.

Beneficence —Requires that the procedure be provided with the intent of doing good for the patient(s) (and participants) involved. This demands that health care providers develop and maintain skills and knowledge, continually update training, consider individual circumstances, and strive for net benefit.

Non-maleficence —Requires that a procedure does not harm the patient involved or others in society. Infertility specialists operate under the assumption that they are doing no harm or at least minimizing harm by pursuing the greater good. However, because assistive reproductive technologies can have limited success rates and uncertain overall outcomes, the emotional state of the patient may be impacted negatively. In some cases, it is difficult for doctors to successfully apply the 'do no harm principle'.

When is an ethical review required?

Any effort in the health system that is not routine and involves patients or the population served by the health services or programmes or any data concerning them and which is intended for publication must be considered 'health research' and ethical approval is needed before starting by a recognized Research Ethics Committee (REC). The following 12 points of ethics must all be addressed:

Scientific merit —The study must have scientific merit and it is important to know—at least—that the question is also valid. A good track record of doing research in this field is useful, but not sufficient.

Ethics review and approval —Protocols must have been approved in writing by a known REC and/or the ethics committee in the national ministry of health. For international collaborative research, approval is usually required from both of the national RECs.

Informed consent —Each patient or participant in a study must have freely and without pressure agreed to participate or not. This is called 'informed consent' or 'informed refusal'. All participants must be given sufficient information in an understandable manner to allow them to decide (with help from relatives or others if they choose) whether or not to participate. There must be an informed consent form for each participant. For guidelines on information required for informed consent see Box 16.2.

Confidentiality —Individuals have the right for their health data to be kept confidential in research studies as in routine data collection. This must be considered because there may be accidental loss of confidentiality. For example, in a study to test a new human immunodeficiency virus (HIV) vaccine all potential participants would first be screened for HIV status. This information must under all circumstances be kept fully confidential.

Risk and benefits —Any research study exposes participants to some measure of risk or discomfort. The risks that participants incur must be in proportion to the potential benefits of the study—most people will find it acceptable to find out about their health status if this is in the context of research on a new drug for treatment or prevention. It is the duty of RECs to ensure a good balance between risks and benefits—this may often be difficult for non-specialists to assess.

Incentives for participation in research —Acceptable reimbursements for research participants can include financial support for travel, food and refreshment, and perhaps money to replace income lost due to the investigation. These are to compensate for costs incurred in participating in the study. Some studies also offer incentives (e.g. small gadgets and even money in excess of what is needed to pay for transport) to encourage people to participate or remain in the study. Incentives should be small enough that people feel free to refuse participate. Large benefits compared to the participants' normal incomes are unethical. They are undue incentives which can appear to be bribe.

Supervision and data safety and monitoring —Research into new interventions, drugs or technologies is normally subject to stringent regulations and standards, one of which is for an independent group of experts to monitor and judge throughout the study period whether they are safe and effective. This group, often called the Data Safety and Monitoring Board (DSMB), is an important safeguard for participants in the studies and certainly should be in place in all drug trials.

Feedback —Participants in studies and their families have a right to know the results of studies in which they participate. Feedback to the participants is too often overlooked. It is good practice to check that all protocols provide for feedback in an understandable manner. Researchers need to offer feedback and acknowledge participants in publications and in public and community meetings.

International studies —Many intervention and drug trials and large research studies in low- and middle-income countries (LMICs) are funded and conducted by institutions based in more developed countries. There is a risk that people in LMICs can be 'used' for research because it may be cheaper or quicker to do research there than in wealthier countries. It is important to seek advice and guidance before collaborating as a partner with international health research organizations and projects.

Individual and community consent —In population-based research, it is often not clear who can give consent for the study, such as participant, family, or husband in some countries, or community chief or district manager:

- Study participants should give informed consent based on their understanding of the full information provided by the researchers.
- At community level, local authorities (e.g. chiefs, village or cell leaders, council chairpersons) must be informed about the research and give their approval for the study to go ahead. However, participation is ultimately decided by individuals under the principle of autonomy. Leaders can support research taking place in their jurisdiction, but not give consent on behalf of others.

Community contracting —Institutions engaging in large-scale international research may have resources much larger than those of the communities in which they work. Some of this may be used to offer assistance, or to set up buildings and even roads and communications, or to train people who can then help with the study. These may provide real benefits to the community long after the study has finished. Local authorities and district health management teams can help by specifying what they and communities will expect in a 'community contract' agreed with researchers and vice versa. Standard guidelines may not be available for such community contracting. Many large-scale research projects, especially in case of product development and economic gain, should set up community contracts before the study starts.

Post-trial treatment —Post-trial treatment should be agreed before any formal approval is granted. If a new drug is tested and found effective, will participants be entitled to continue to receive the new drug when the trial finishes? Should the placebo group(s) also receive the drug? Should these be provided free and if so, for how long? The pharmaceutical company may be required to continue providing free effective treatment after completing such trials. If research leads to an effective treatment many countries require the pharmaceutical companies to continue treatments for all study participants for a stated period, such as five years. Post-trial treatment should be agreed before formal approval is granted.

Index